B. Marincek · P. R. Ros · M. Reiser · M. E. Baker (Eds.)

Multislice CT: A Practical Guide

Springer

Berlin
Heidelberg
New York
Barcelona
Hong Kong
London
Milan
Paris
Singapore
Tokyo

B. Marincek · P. R. Ros · M. Reiser
M. E. Baker (Eds.)

Multislice CT:
A Practical Guide

**Proceedings of the 5th International
SOMATOM CT Scientific User Conference
Zurich, June 2000**

With 134 Figures and 15 Tables

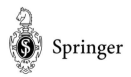 Springer

Borut Marincek, M. D.

Professor and Chairman
University Hospital
Institute of Diagnostic Radiology
Rämistrasse 100
CH-8091 Zürich

Pablo R. Ros, M. D., MPH

Vice Chairman, Operations & Planning
Director, Partners Radiology
Professor of Radiology
Harvard Medical School
Brigham and Women's Hospital
75 Francis Street
Boston, MA 02115 / USA

Maximilian Reiser, M. D.

Professor and Chairman
Department of Clinical Radiology
Klinikum Grosshadern
Ludwig Maximilians-University
Marchioninistrasse 15
D-81377 Munich

Mark E. Baker, M. D.

Head, Section of Abdominal Imaging
Division of Radiology
The Cleveland Clinic Foundation
9500 Euclid Ave.
Cleveland, OH 44195 / USA

ISBN   3-540-41116-X Springer-Verlag Berlin Heidelberg New York

Die Deutsche Bibliothek - CIP-Einheitsaufnahme

Multislice CT - a practical guide : proceedings of th e 5th
International SOMATOM CT Scientific User Conference, Zürich, June 2000
/ ed.: Borut Marincek .... – Berlin ; Heidelberg ; New York ;
Barcelona ; Hong Kong ; London ; Milan ; Paris ; Singapore ; Tokyo :
Springer, 2001
     ISBN 3-540-41116-X

Springer-Verlag Berlin Heidelberg New York
is a member of BertelmannSpringer Science+Business Media GmbH
© Springer-Verlag Berlin Heidelberg 2001
Printed in Germany

The use of general descriptive names, registered names, trademarks, etc. in this publication
does not imply, even in the absence of a specific statement, that such names are exempt from
the relevant protective laws and regulations and therefore free for general use.

Product liability: The publisher cannot guarantee the accuracy of any information about
dosage and application contained in this book. In every individual case the user must check
such information by consulting the relevant literature.

Cover design: design & production GmbH, Heidelberg
Typesetting: cicero Lasersatz, Dinkelscherben
Printed on acid-free paper   –   SPIN: 10784745   18/3130   5 4 3 2 1 0

Preface

Until recently, CT scanner performance was limited by a series of compromises. With single-detector scanners, one cannot select thin collimation and still maintain the required extent of volumetric coverage. Slow scans cause motion artifacts that impair image quality. The introduction of multidetector CT technology, however, has revolutionized the field. Currently multidetector, multislice CT scanners acquire up to four channels of data from interweaving spirals. The minimum gantry rotation period is as low as half of a second. This increased scan speed allows for thinner collimation and thus higher longitudinal or z-axis resolution in comparison with single-detector CT.

The improved image quality with multidetector technology leads to new applications of CT, particularly in cardiac, vascular, and abdominal imaging. On-going clinical studies are evaluating the suitability of this new imaging tool for non-invasive screening and diagnosis of coronary artery disease. A particular advantage to the increased scan speed in vascular imaging is the ability to cut intravenous contrast dosage and still maintain peak enhancement throughout the entire acquisition. Thin-section, multiphasic CT acquisition during optimal arterial-phase and venous-phase enhancement significantly improves the accuracy for small lesion and vessel detection, and enhances overall classification of abdominal neoplasms. On the other hand, the increasingly large volume data sets force to new ways of looking at, presenting, storing, and transferring images. Networking and two- and three dimensional data processing are the key words. These challenges have been met and have already been rapidly transferred by radiologists to the clinical environment to improve diagnosis and patient care.

In an effort to demonstrate the clinical advantages of multislice CT several groups of experts have been invited to the 5th SOMATOM CT Scientific User Conference. The increasing international ambiance of this traditional meeting is reflected in the joint hosting of four well known universities in Europe and the USA. The conference was held in Zurich in mid June 2000 under the auspices of the University Hospital Zurich, the Klinikum Grosshadern, Munich, the Brigham and Women's Hospital, Boston, and The Cleveland Clinic Foundation, Ohio.

The experiences presented at the meeting with the newest member of the SOMATOM family, the "SOMATOM Volume Zoom", are collected in this book. The contributions will familiarize the practitioner with relevant aspects of multislice CT. A thorough understanding of this new technology is a prerequsite to fully exploit its diagnostic potential.

We would like to thank all authors for their enthusiasm and superb work. The excellent secretarial work of Madeleine Meyer and the professional help of the editorial team at Springer-Verlag is also gratefully acknowledged.

Zurich, July 2000   BORUT MARINCEK, Zurich, Switzerland
                           MAXIMILIAN REISER, Munich, Germany
                           PABLO R. ROS, Boston, USA
                           MARK E. BAKER, Ohio, USA

Contents

I Technical Aspects of Multislice Computed Tomography

Spiral and Multislice Computed Tomography Scanning:
Physical Principles that Inform Protocol Development
STEVEN E. SELTZER 3

Multislice Scanning with the SOMATOM Volume Zoom
THOMAS H. FLOHR, KLAUS KLINGENBECK-REGN,
BERND OHNESORGE, STEFAN SCHALLER 7

What is Changed in Contrast Medium Injection
when Using High-Resolution Multislice Computed Tomography?
ROBERTO PASSARIELLO, CARLO CATALANO, FEDERICA PEDICONI,
ROBERTO BRILLO 22

Computer Modeling Approach to Contrast Medium Administration and Scan Timing for Multislice Computed Tomography
KYONGTAE T. BAE, JAY P. HEIKEN 28

Three-Dimensional Imaging and Virtual Reality Applications of
Multislice Computed Tomography
SIMON WILDERMUTH, NINOSLAV TEODOROVIC,
PAUL R. HILFIKER, BORUT MARINCEK 37

II Multislice Computed Tomography in Neuroradiology

Intracranial and Cervical Three-Dimensional Computed
Tomography Angiography Using a Multislice Computed
Tomography System: Initial Clinical Experience
YUKUNORI KOROGI, KAZUHIRO YOSHIZUMI,
YOSHIHARU NAKAYAMA, MASATAKA KADOTA,
MUTSUMASA TAKAHASHI 59

Multislice Spiral Computed Tomography of the Skull Base
ULRICH BAUM, BERND TOMANDL, MICHAEL LELL, MATTHIAS
DUETSCH, KNUT EBERHARDT, HOLGER GREESS, WERNER BAUTZ 65

III Cardiovascular Multislice Computed Tomography

Cardiac Imaging with Multislice Computed Tomography Scan
and Reconstruction Principles and Quality Assurance
WILLI A. KALENDER, STEFAN ULZHEIMER, MARC KACHELRIESS   79

The Potential of Cardio-Computed Tomography
ALEXANDER V. SMEKAL   90

Coronary Atherosclerosis in Multislice Computed Tomography
CHRISTOPH R. BECKER, BERND M. OHNESORGE,
U. JOSEPH SCHOEPF, MAXIMILIAN F. REISER   98

Coronary Computed Tomography Angiography Using Multislice
Computed Tomography: Pitfalls and Potential
MALTE L. BAHNER, J. M. BOESE 111

Cardiac Multislice Computed Tomography:
Screening and Diagnosis of Chronic Heart Disease
ANDREAS F. KOPP, STEPHEN SCHRÖDER, AXEL KÜTTNER,
CHRISTIAN GEORG, BERND OHNESORGE, CLAUS D. CLAUSSEN . 118

Real Time Visualization of Volume Data:
Applications in Computed Tomography Angiography
ELLIOT K. FISHMAN 125

Fast High-Resolution Computed Tomography Angiography of
Peripheral Vessels
CARLO CATALANO, ANDREA GROSSI, ALESSANDRO NAPOLI,
FRANCESCO FRAIOLI 134

IV Multislice Computed Tomography Applications in the Chest

Multislice Computed Tomography of the Lung Parenchyma
MATHIAS PROKOP 145

Multisclice CT in Pulmonary Embolism
U. JOSEPH SCHOEPF 157

The Radiologist's Role in Radiation Exposure
during Chest Computed Tomography
PETER VOCK, ULRIKE BREHMER 169

V Multislice Computed Tomography Applications in the Abdomen

Multidetector, Multislice Spiral Computed Tomography
of the Abdomen: Quo Vadis
MARK E. BAKER, BRIAN R. HERTS, WILLIAM T. DAVROS 179

Multislice Computed Tomography of the Urinary Tract
STUART G. SILVERMAN 188

Application of Multislice Computed Tomography
in Liver and Pancreas
HOON JI, PABLO R. ROS 195

Virtual Endoscopy
DIDIER BIELEN, DIRK VANBECKEVOORT, MAARTEN THOMEER,
MARC PEETERS 204

Multislice Computed Tomography Colonography:
Technique Optimization
ANDREA LAGHI, VALERIA PANEBIANCO, CARLO CATALANO,
RICCARDO IANNACCONE, FILIPPO G. ASSAEL, SANTE IORI,
ROBERTO PASSARIELLO 216

Subject Index 227

List of Contributors

F. G. Assael
Department of Radiology, University of Rome "La Sapienza",
Viale Regina Elena 324, 00161 Rome, Italy

K. T. Bae
Department of Radiology, Mallinckrodt Institute of Radiology,
510 South Kingshighway Boulevard, St. Louis, MO 63110 USA

M. L. Bahner
Abt. Onkologische Diagnostik und Therapie, Deutsches Krebs-
forschungszentrum, Im Neuenheimer Feld 280, 69120 Heidelberg,
Germany

M. E. Baker
Division of Radiology, The Cleveland Clinic Foundation,
9500 Euclid Avenue, Cleveland OH 44195, USA

U. Baum
Institute of Diagnostic Radiology, Friedrich-Alexander-
University Erlangen-Nuremberg, Maximiliansplatz 1,
91054 Erlangen, Germany

W. Bautz
Institute of Diagnostic Radiology, Friedrich-Alexander-
University Erlangen-Nuremberg, Maximiliansplatz 1,
91054 Erlangen, Germany

C. R. Becker
Department of Clinical Radiology, Ludwig-Maximilians-
University, Klinikum Grosshadern, Marchioninistrasse 15,
81377 Munich, Germany

D. Bielen
Department of Radiology, University Hospital KU Leuven,
Herestraat 49, 3000 Leuven, Belgium

J. M. Boese
   Abt. Onkologische Diagnostik und Therapie,
   Deutsches Krebsforschungszentrum, Im Neuenheimer Feld 280,
   69120 Heidelberg, Germany

U. Brehmer
   Institute of Diagnostic Radiology, Inselspital Bern,
   Freiburgstrasse, 3010 Bern, Switzerland

C. Catalano
   Department of Radiology, University of Rome "La Sapienza",
   Viale Regina Elena 324, 00161 Rome, Italy

C. D. Claussen
   Abt. für Radiologische Diagnostik,
   Universitätsklinikum Tübingen, Hoppe-Seyler-Strasse 3,
   72076 Tübingen, Germany

W. T. Davros
   Division of Radiology, The Cleveland Clinic Foundation,
   9500 Euclid Avenue, Cleveland OH 44195, USA

M. Duetsch
   Division of Neurology, Friedrich-Alexander-University Erlangen-
   Nuremberg, Schwabachanlage 6, 91054 Erlangen, Germany

K. Eberhardt
   Division of Neurology, Friedrich-Alexander-University
   Erlangen-Nuremberg, Schwabachanlage 6, 91054 Erlangen,
   Germany

E. K. Fishman
   Department of Radiology and Radiological Science,
   Johns Hopkins University School of Medicine,
   601 North Caroline Street, Baltimore, MD 21287, USA

Th. Flohr
   Department of Computed Tomography, Siemens Medical
   Engineering, Siemensstrasse 1, 91301 Forchheim, Germany

F. Fraioli
   Department of Radiology, University of Rome "La Sapienza",
   Viale Regina Elena 324, 00161 Rome, Italy

C. George
   Abt. für Radiologische Diagnostik, Universitätsklinikum
   Tübingen, Hoppe-Seyler-Strasse 3, 72076 Tübingen,
   Germany

H. Greess
Institute of Diagnostic Radiology, Friedrich-Alexander-University Erlangen-Nuremberg, Maximiliansplatz 1, 91054 Erlangen, Germany

A. Grossi
Department of Radiology, University of Rome "La Sapienza", Viale Regina Elena 324, 00161 Rome, Italy

J. P. Heiken
Department of Radiology, Mallinckrodt Institute of Radiology, 510 South Kingshighway Boulevard, St. Louis, MO 63110 USA

B. R. Herts
Division of Radiology, The Cleveland Clinic Foundation, 9500 Euclid Avenue, Cleveland OH 44195, USA

P. R. Hilfiker
Institute of Diagnostic Radiology, University Hospital, Rämistrasse 100, 8091 Zurich, Switzerland

R. Ianinaccone
Department of Radiology, University of Rome "La Sapienza", Viale Regina Elena 324, 00161 Rome, Italy

S. Iori
Department of Radiology, University of Rome "La Sapienza", Viale Regina Elena 324, 00161 Rome, Italy

H. Ji
Department of Radiology, Brigham and Women's Hospital, 75 Francis Street, Boston, MA 02115, USA

M. Kachelries
Institute of Medical Physics (IMP), University Erlangen, Krankenhausstrasse 12, 91054 Erlangen, Germany

M. Kadota
Department of Radiology, Kumamoto University School of Medicine, 1-1-1 Honjo, Kumamoto 860-8556, Japan

W. A. Kalender
Institute of Medical Physics (IMP), University Erlangen, Krankenhausstrasse 12, 91054 Erlangen, Germany

K. Klingenbeck-Regn
Department of Computed Tomography, Siemens Medical Engineering, Siemensstrasse 1, 91301 Forchheim, Germany

A. F. Kopp
Abt. für Radiologische Diagnostik, Universitätsklinikum
Tübingen, Hoppe-Seyler-Strasse 3, 72076 Tübingen,
Germany

Y. Korogi
Department of Radiology, Kumamoto University School of
Medicine, 1-1-1 Honjo, Kumamoto 860-8556, Japan

A. Kuettner
Abt. für Radiologische Diagnostik, Universitätsklinikum
Tübingen, Hoppe-Seyler-Strasse 3, 72076 Tübingen,
Germany

A. Laghi
Department of Radiology, University of Rome "La Sapienza",
Viale Regina Elena 324, 00161 Rome, Italy

M. Lell
Institute of Diagnostic Radiology, Friedrich-Alexander-
University Erlangen-Nuremberg, Maximiliansplatz 1,
91054 Erlangen, Germany

B. Marincek
Institute of Diagnostic Radiology, University Hospital Zurich,
Rämistrasse 100, 8091 Zurich, Switzerland

Y. Nakayama
Department of Radiology, Kumamoto University School of
Medicine, 1-1-1 Honjo, Kumamoto 860-8556, Japan

A. Napoli
Department of Radiology, University of Rome "La Sapienza",
Viale Regina Elena 324, 00161 Rome, Italy

B. M. Ohnesorge
Department of Clinical Radiology, Ludwig-Maximilians-
University, Klinikum Grosshadern, Marchioninistrasse 15,
81377 Munich, Germany

B. Ohnesorge
Department of Computed Tomography, Siemens Medical
Engineering, Siemensstrasse 1, 91301 Forchheim, Germany

V. Panebianco
Department of Radiology, University of Rome "La Sapienza",
Viale Regina Elena 324, 00161 Rome, Italy

R. PASSARIELLO
Department of Radiology, University of Rome "La Sapienza",
Viale Regina Elena 324, 00161 Rome, Italy

M. PEETERS
Department of Radiology, University Hospital KU Leuven,
Herestraat 49, 3000 Leuven, Belgium

M. PROKOP
Department of Diagnostic Radiology, Vienna General Hospital
(AKH Wien), Währinger Gürtel 18–20, 1090 Vienna, Austria

M. F. REISER
Department of Clinical Radiology, Ludwig-Maximilians-
University, Klinikum Grosshadern, Marchioninistrasse 15,
81377 Munich, Germany

P. R. Ros
Department of Radiology, Brigham and Women's Hospital,
75 Francis Street, Boston, MA 02115, USA

B. SCHALLER
Department of Computed Tomography, Siemens Medical
Engineering, Siemensstrasse 1, 91301 Forchheim, Germany

U. J. SCHOEPF
Department of Clinical Radiology, Ludwig-Maximilians-
University, Klinikum Grosshadern, Marchioninistrasse 15,
81377 Munich, Germany

S. SCHROEDER
Abt. für Radiologische Diagnostik, Universitätsklinikum
Tübingen, Hoppe-Seyler-Strasse 3, 72076 Tübingen,
Germany

S. E. SELTZER
Department of Radiology, Brigham and Women's Hospital,
75 Francis Street, Boston, MA 02115, USA

S. G. SILVERMAN
Department of Radiology, Brigham and Women's Hospital,
75 Francis Street, Boston, MA 02115, USA

M. TAKAHASHI
Department of Radiology, Kumamoto University School of
Medicine, 1-1-1 Honjo, Kumamoto 860-8556, Japan

N. Teodorovic
   Institute of Diagnostic Radiology, University Hospital,
   Rämistrasse 100, 8091 Zurich, Switzerland

M. Thomeer
   Department of Radiology, University Hospital KU Leuven,
   Herestraat 49, 3000 Leuven, Belgium

B. Tomandl
   Division of Neuroradiology, Friedrich-Alexander-University
   Erlangen-Nuremberg, Schwabachanlage 6, 91054 Erlangen,
   Germany

S. Ulzheimer
   Institute of Medical Physics (IMP), University Erlangen,
   Krankenhausstrasse 12, 91054 Erlangen, Germany

D. Vanbeckevoort
   Department of Radiology, University Hospital KU Leuven,
   Herestraat 49, 3000 Leuven, Belgium

P. Vock
   Institute of Diagnostic Radiology, Inselspital Bern,
   Freiburgstrasse, 3010 Bern, Switzerland

A. von Smekal
   Institute of Diagnostic Radiology, University Hospital,
   Rämistrasse 100, 8091 Zurich, Switzerland

S. Wildermuth
   Center for Bioinformatics, NASA Ames Research Center,
   Moffett Field, CA 94035, USA

K. Yoshizumi
   Department of Radiology, Kumamoto University School of
   Medicine, 1-1-1 Honjo, Kumamoto 860-8556, Japan

I Technical Aspects
of Multislice Computed Tomography

Spiral and Multislice Computed Tomography Scanning: Physical Principles that Inform Protocol Development

Steven E. Seltzer

Abstract. Spiral computed tomography affords the user a wide variety of selectable technical parameters. Despite more than 10 years of experience with this technique and its more advanced cousin, multislice CT, there is little international agreement to the optimum technical parameters to use. No single combination of these parameters is ideal for every indication. Specifically, there will always be trade-offs between radiation dose, image noise, image sharpness, and the amount of region coverage. The goal of this paper is to help the practitioner understand the physical principles that contribute to CT image quality and allow the design of optimal protocols for a variety of clinical situations.

Measures of Image Quality in Spiral/Multislice Computed Tomography

While a full discussion of the appropriate measures of image quality is well beyond the scope of this short article, a simplified listing of key parameters is useful for the practitioner. These include:

Image Noise

Random pixel-to-pixel variations in measured computed tomography (CT) attenuation coefficients are the result of stochastic variations in CT image production. This variability is due to the finite number of X-ray photons used to create the image itself. The amount of noise present is inversely proportional to the square root of the number of photons used to produce the image. When conspicuous, noise manifests itself as a "grainy" character to the image itself and can obscure the detection of low-contrast objects.

Radiation Dose

From the preceding discussion, it is clear that the amount of noise can be affected directly by the radiation dose. Therefore, a balance must be struck between the desire to reduce image noise and the risks of radiation exposure to the patient. A typical clinically useful X-ray tube output (for example, 250 mAs at 120 kVp) results in a 3-to-5 rad exposure to the patient from each slice.

Image Sharpness

In the plane of the image slice, several factors affect the perceived sharpness of the CT image. Perhaps the most important of these is the so-called partial volume averaging effect. As is well known, if more than one tissue type is included in the imaging voxel, the resulting measured attenuation coefficient is the weighted average of the two types in the proportion of the slice thickness that they occupy.

The visual impact of this averaging is a decrease in the perceived sharpness of the edges of structures and a decrease in the conspicuity of small high-contrast objects (smaller than the effective slice thickness). The effective slice thickness can also be influenced by the table feed speed and the interpolation algorithm used for image reconstruction. That is, slower feed speeds and algorithms based on 180° linear interpretation tend to have thinner nominal slices.

In addition, the reconstruction kernel selected can affect sharpness. For instance, edge-enhancing algorithms increase perceived sharpness (but also increase the visibility of random variations or noise). In the Z-axis, the sharpness of multi-planar reconstruction is affected by the slice thickness and the degree of overlap from one slice to the next.

Coverage

The amount of tissue covered in a spiral CT acquisition is a function of the table feed speed and the duration of the exposure.

User-Selectable Parameters

Table 1 lists the common user-selectable parameters in a spiral CT examination. Six such factors are common to both spiral and conventional imaging protocols, while four are specific to spiral protocols themselves.

Table 1. User-selectable parameters

Common to spiral and conventional protocols
– kVp
– mA
– Gantry rotation speed
– Slice thickness
– Reconstruction algorithm
– Contrast delivery parameters
Amount/volume
Rate
Phases
Delay
Specific to Spiral Protocols
– Table feed speed (pitch)
– Algorithm 360/180°
– Exposure duration
– Reconstruction increment

Table 2. Impact of technical parameters on spiral image quality

Parameter	Noise	Sharpness
Slice thickness-thinner	Increase	Increase
Table feed speed faster	Constant	Decrease
mA-increase	Decrease	Constant
KVP-increase	No sign Δ	No sign Δ
Reconstruction alogo-sharper	Increase	Increase
Reconstruction increment-finer	Constant	Increase in z-axis

KVP, peak kilovoltage of the X-ray tube

As can be seen from the preceding discussion, the selection of many of these parameters involves the operator making a trade-off of two critical elements of image quality. Most commonly, this trade-off is between the amount of noise and the amount of sharpness in the image. For example, decreasing the effective slice thickness can increase sharpness (through decreasing the amount of partial volume averaging present) but at the same time increase the amount of noise in the image (by reducing the number of photons used).

Similarly, the use of a sharper reconstruction kernel can improve sharpness but will increase the conspicuity of the perceived noise. Table 2 summarizes the impact on noise and sharpness of six common user-selectable parameters. The table emphasizes the fact that there is no single optimal combination of these parameters that both minimizes noise and increases sharpness.

Rational Protocol Development

The user can maximize the quality of imaging protocols by segregating studies into three major categories. For survey studies (such as the evaluation of trauma or the search for the extent of disease in an oncologic patient), the critical element that must not be sacrificed is the adequate coverage of the entire region of interest. Typically, relatively thick slices (5–7 mm) are used with a table feed speed that is adequate to cover the entire region of interest in a single breath hold. These relatively long exposures place a cap on the tube current (hence also determining radiation dose and image noise) that can be utilized. In modern systems, however, the tube current for a 30–50 s exposure can be greater than 250–300 mA. Therefore, one should employ the minimum radiation dose required to provide adequate visualization of the desired structures.

In focused studies, one generally uses thinner slices (1–3 mm) and needs only relatively slow table feed speeds. Examples of this type of study would be the search for a small adrenal gland nodule or a small pancreatic mass. Typically, images can be acquired easily in a single breath hold in milliamp values adequate to provide excellent detail and limited noise.

In CT angiography, the user is called upon to accomplish two contradictory goals. That is, it is necessary to depict small blood vessels down to a size of 1 mm or 2 mm, while at the same time covering a large area of the body (such as the thoracoabdominal aorta). For this type of study, one typically utilizes a combination of thin slices (1–3 mm) with a rapid table feed speed. The thinking is that if one starts with a relatively thin slice, one can then tolerate the moderate amount of broadening of effective slice thickness that accrues from the faster feed speed in order to have adequate coverage. Z-axis resolution for three-dimensional and multi-planar reconstruction is optimized by having a high degree of overlap of adjacent slices (typically a 1-mm or 2-mm table increment).

Multislice Scanners

The advent of multislice CT represents an enormous technical advance and will be discussed thoroughly in other papers in this series. By acquiring multiple slices simultaneously, the user can achieve shorter data acquisition times, greater coverage, and improved sharpness (via use of thinner slices), or can mix and match elements of each of these advantages.

In addition, because one can reconstruct slices with a variety of thicknesses after the image data has been acquired, the operator has yet an additional degree of freedom in prescribing the examination protocol. This permits the distinction between survey and focused studies to be de-emphasized. This is true because a broad coverage study can be obtained with relatively thick slices followed by images from a defined area of interest with thinner slices without the need to re-expose the patient.

For better or worse, the flexibility afforded by multislice CT systems introduces even more options for the operator. This flexibility makes it more critical than ever for the operator to be familiar with the physical principles of spiral CT scanning and the trade-offs that exist amongst technical parameters and image quality. Armed with this knowledge, optimal protocols can be designed and optimum choices made (Table 1 and Table 2).

Suggested Reading

1. Barnes GT, Lakshminarayan AV(1998) Conventional and spiral computed tomography: physical principles and image quality considerations. In: Lee JKT, Stanley RI, Sagel SS, Heiken JP (eds) Computed body tomography with MRI correlation. Lippincott-Raven, Philadelphia pp 1–20
2. Kalender WA, Scissler W, Klotz E, Vock P (1990) Spiral volumetric CT with single-breath-hold technique, continuous transport, and continuous scanner rotation. Radiology 176:181–183
3. Rigauts H, Marchal G, Baert AL, Hupke R (1990) Initial experience with volume CT scanning. J Comput Assist Tomogr 14:675–682
4. Fishman EK, Jeffrey Jr RB (eds) (1995) Spiral CT: principles, techniques and clinical applications. Raven Press, New York
5. Kalender WA, Polacin A (1991) Physical performance characteristics of spiral CT scanning. Med Phys 18:910–915
6. Polacin A, Kalender WA, Marchal G (1992) Evaluation of section sensitivity profiles and image noise in spiral CT. Radiology 185:29–35
7. Brink JA, Heiken JP, Balfe DM, et al. (1992) Spiral CT: decreased spatial resolution in vivo to broadening of section-sensitivity profile. Radiology 185:469–474

Multislice CT Scanning with the SOMATOM Volume Zoom

THOMAS H. FLOHR, KLAUS KLINGENBECK-REGN, BERND OHNESORGE, STEFAN SCHALLER

Introduction

With the advent of slip ring technology, continuous rotation of the measurement system and continuous data acquisition became possible. Together with continuous table motion during data acquisition, spiral imaging development and introduction into clinical practice in the early 1990s was made possible [1, 2].

For the first time, spiral computed tomography (CT) allowed for the acquisition of continuous volume data. As such, spiral CT paved the way for CT angiography (CTA) to become successful in clinical routine. The limitation of spiral CT with single slice scanners is the limited volume coverage with thin slices. Isotropic resolution in a volume remained a dream apart from some very special applications [3].

In this respect, the introduction of fast multislice scanners at the 1998 annual meeting of the Radiological Society of North America (RSNA) is a real quantum leap towards isotropic volume imaging. A logical consequence is a transition from the traditional way of viewing the information in a transaxial fashion to automated and integrated methods of volumetric viewing as the primary step to diagnosis. The SOMATOM Volume Zoom has been designed to optimally support those clinical requirements in terms of acquisition, image quality, and handling of the large, isotropic data sets. In this paper, we will cover some of the basic design considerations and the major advantages for clinical applications [4].

Design Considerations

When considering the design of a multislice CT (MSCT) scanner, it is helpful and instructive to consider the following example: scanning of the thorax with narrow collimation, such as beams of 1-mm thickness within an average breath hold time of 25 s. The fastest single slice scanner, available in 1995, the SOMATOM Plus 4 with 0.75 s rotation time could cover 50 mm of anatomy in the given time (Fig. 1a) with a standard pitch of 1.5. The goal to cover 300 mm of anatomy is off by a factor of six.

By adding the simultaneous read out of four 1-mm slices, considerable improvements can be achieved but still the desired coverage is off by a factor of 1.5 (6/4). Adding a second element, the faster rotation of 0.5 s finally achieves the goal. Both elements, simultaneous read out of four slices and the fast rotation of 0.5 s need to be combined [4] to realize such an application (Fig. 1b). Further-

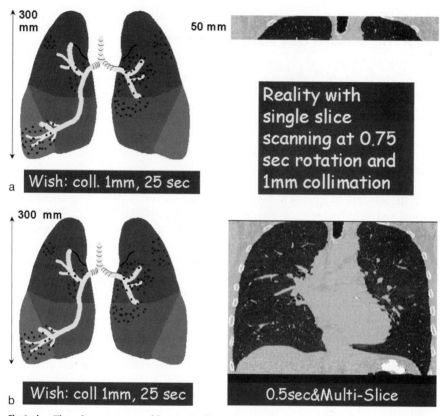

Fig. 1a, b. a The volume coverage of fast single slice scanners with a beam collimation of 1 mm is severely limited. **b** Multislice acquisition and fast rotation of 0.5 s are needed to achieve the volume coverage with 1-mm collimation

more, the fast rotation in combination with dedicated scan and reconstruction techniques is the key to image the heart anatomy free of motion (Fig. 2). Cardiac CT scanning [5] will be considered in a separate section.

With those technical innovations, the general performance of fast multislice scanners is improved significantly by a factor of eight (four slices in 0.5 s) as related to previous standards of single slice scanners with 1.0 s per image. Such an increased performance can be utilized in several ways: isotropic imaging of anatomical volumes, imaging of long volumes within practical scan times and imaging of anatomical volumes in very short scan times. In practice, the diagnostic intention will define how such improved performance is utilized clinically.

Basically, MSCT scanning is nothing else than acquiring four slices during one rotation instead of performing four single slice acquisitions with table feed in between (Fig. 3). However, the practical application of the technique requires the adaptation of the collimation to the needs of the examination under consideration. Therefore, the detector design must be more elaborate than just stacking four detector banks one after the other in an axial direction.

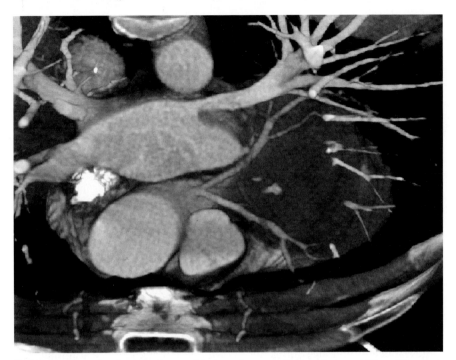

Fig. 2. Three-dimensional-rendered view of the heart from a multislice spiral acquisition with optimized temporal resolution

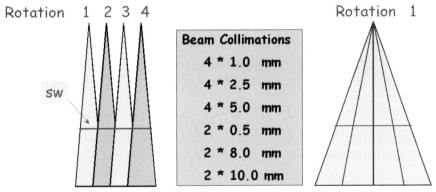

Fig. 3. Simultaneous acquisition of multiple slices during a single rotation of the computed tomography scanner relative to consecutive acquisitions with a single slice scanner

For the SOMATOM Volume Zoom, the adaptive array detector [4] has been developed. This solution maximizes the dose efficiency, since a minimum number of separate detector elements is combined in axial direction to read out the four slice combinations which are shown in Figure 4. Consequently, the number of dead spaces between detector rows is minimized, and the geometric efficiency is maximized.

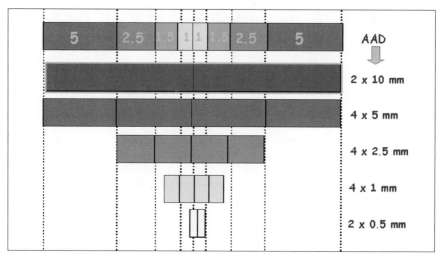

Fig. 4. The principle of the adaptive array detector (AAD). Various slice combinations can be generated by varying the beam collimation and the combination of detector signals during read-out

For spiral imaging, the extended sampling patterns of MSCT allow the realization of new concepts and algorithms not known before in single slice scanning. The key elements for this are new, in general, nonlinear spiral algorithms which are described elsewhere in detail [6, 7].

Here we summarize the major benefits for clinical application:

1. Slice sensitivity profiles, which are independent of pitch. As a result, isotropic resolution can be maintained at any table speed.
2. Dose and image noise independent on pitch.
3. Free selection of pitch between 1 and 8.
4. No noise enhancement over sequential images and corresponding dose savings between 30% and 40%.
5. Dedicated cardiac spiral algorithms.

In the following section, we will work out the major advantages of the above issues in clinical applications.

Major Advantages of MSCT

Transaxial MSCT also benefits from multislice acquisition in terms of speed and flexibility. As an example, the whole brain can be scanned with 4 x 5-mm sections in less than 10 s. Another example is scanning of the base of the skull with the 4 x 1-mm collimator setting to avoid partial volume artifacts. Fusion of the thin cuts to 4-mm wide slices then restores low noise images for soft tissue diagnosis free of streak artifacts [4]. However, the real power of MSCT becomes evident in spiral imaging, which we will concentrate on next.

Isotropic Imaging

A key benefit is the ability of MSCT to scan anatomical volumes with isotropic resolution. Previously, there was quite some mismatch between a slice thickness of 5 mm and an in-plane resolution of about 1 mm, typical values for an abdominal scan (Fig. 5). Employing fast rotation and fast table motion, narrow collimated scans can cover the desired anatomy within practical times and with isotropic resolution. A typical technique is, for example, 4 x 1-mm beam collimation, 0.5 s rotation, and a pitch of 7.3 to cover 400 mm in 27 s. Such capabilities then also question our traditional way of viewing the data in a transaxial fashion. Given isotropy, it is more logical and might be more efficient to primarily view longitudinally with coronal and sagittal multi-planar reformations (MPRs; Fig. 6). Similarly, other methods of 3D viewing, maximum intensity projections (MIPs) and volume renderings (VRs), are likely to change their traditional role of methods for post-processing to become automated and integrated tools for primary diagnosis. Some applications are shown in Figures 7 and 8. The underlying

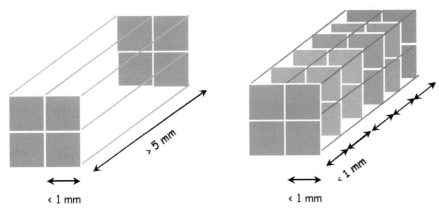

Fig. 5. Multislice scanning and fast rotation allows the transition to isotropic resolution

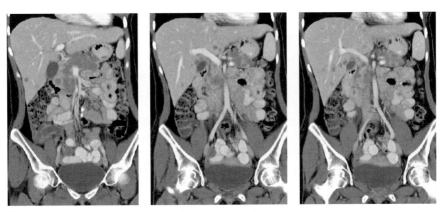

Fig. 6. Volume viewing in terms of coronal multi-planar reformations

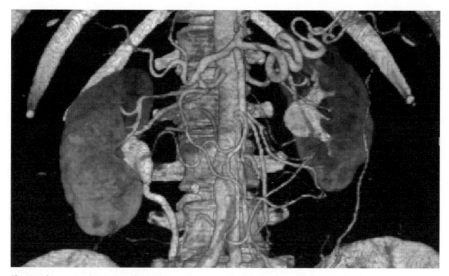

Fig. 7. Volume viewing using three-dimensional rendering

theme is isotropic resolution of the data and, related to this, the freedom to navigate through the volume.

Presently, the large amount of volumetric data, as a consequence of isotropy, is necessarily the most disputed issue. Automation and integration of 3D processing into the examination protocols with proper settings for visualization and evaluation are very demanding requirements for clinical research. The workflow on the SOMATOM Volume Zoom has been prepared for such demands by providing two PC-based stations, which are linked by a shared data base. This allows instant access of the data from both consoles, thereby eliminating the transfer times via networks.

The various functionalities, available under the Syngo platform, can be configured and distributed amongst the consoles to tailor to the specific workflow needs of routine applications. For more time consuming, advanced 3D process-

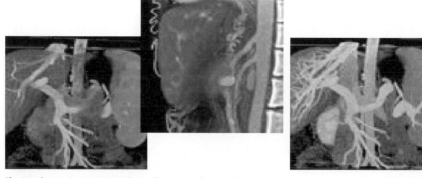

Fig. 8. Volume viewing using three-dimensional rendering

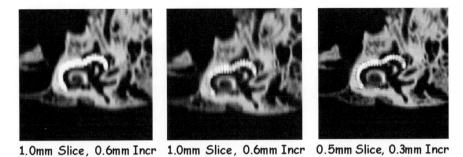

1.0mm Slice, 0.6mm Incr   1.0mm Slice, 0.6mm Incr   0.5mm Slice, 0.3mm Incr
17 lp/cm   22 lp/cm   22 lp/cm

Fig. 9. High resolution in plane, 20 lp/cm and beyond requires the use of sub-millimeter slices for dedicated applications

Direct Axials

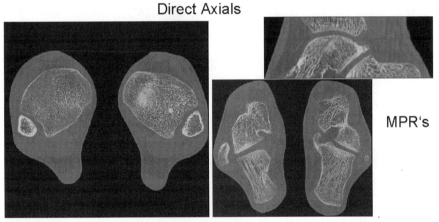

MPR's

Fig. 10. Isotropy at high resolution: a practical example

ing, the 3D Virtuoso workstation is available for powerful volume rendering in real time.

For dedicated applications with high in-plane resolution, isotropy requires the use of sub-millimeter collimation. An example is given in Figure 9 for a phantom with a cochlear implant. Obviously, it is important to match the axial resolution to the desired in-plane resolution for optimized image quality in 3D. Another example is given in Figure 10 for high resolution of joints with the 0.5 mm collimation. The high contrast resolution of corresponding MPRs is visually identical to the image quality in a transaxial representation.

A consequence of the ability to scan anatomical volumes with narrow collimation is the ability to retrieve different information, such as low and high contrast information from the same scan. The underlying reason is that for multislice spiral scanning, the slice width and the collimation are no longer uniquely related. There is much more flexibility and, based on this, new strategies for planning a CT examination can be derived. For example, the data from a scan with 4 x 1-mm collimation can be reconstructed to slices of multiple widths ranging

Slice Width / mm

Collimation / mm	0.5	0.75	1.0	1.25	1.5	2.0	3.0	4.0	5.0	6.0	7.0	8.0	10.0
2*0.5	y	y	y	y	y	y							
4*1.0			y	y	y	y	y	y	y	y	y	y	y
4*2.5							y	y	y	y	y	y	y
4*5.0										y	y	y	y

Fig. 11. Slice widths that can be derived from scanning with given collimator settings

from 1 mm to 10 mm. Figure 11 gives a complete overview for the collimator settings available for the SOMATOM Volume Zoom.

An application of this technique is illustrated in Figure 12. The high resolution lung images and the standard mediastinal images are derived from the same data taken with the 4 x 1-mm collimation [8]. The corresponding reconstruction tasks

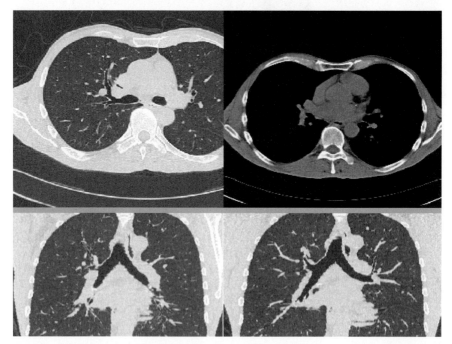

Fig. 12. High and low contrast information from the same scan (combi scan of the SOMATOM Volume Zoom)

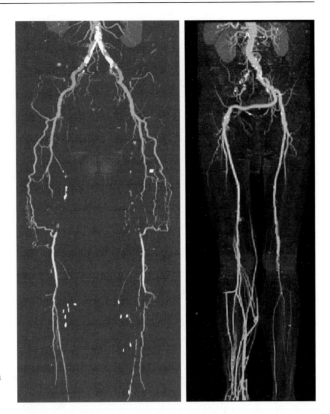

Fig. 13. Computed
tomography angiography
of the legs in a patient with
advanced arteriosclerotic
occlusive disease

can be defined prospectively; the system automatically provides both sets of
images from the same data set. Narrow slices may then be used for further 3D
processing, as discussed earlier.

The ability to scan long volumes is of importance in a variety of other cases,
such as CTA of the extremities (Fig. 13) or CTA of the whole aorta, where it might
be more important to cover a length of a meter and more within a given bolus
time and to compromise on highest axial resolution. With the 4 x 2.5 mm
collimator setting, a maximum table feed of 20 mm per rotation can be achieved.
In combination with the fastest rotation time of 0.5 s, the volume coverage ranges
up to 40 mm/s, which allows for scanning one meter in 25 s. Note that fast
rotation is an important element also for this application; at 0.75 s, the volume
coverage would be 27 mm/s, with a scan time of 38 s.

A third major advantage is to use performance to achieve very short scan times.
A corresponding scan technique is as follows: 4 x 2.5-mm collimation, 0.5 s rotation time, and a pitch of 6.7. Then a typical thorax of 300 mm length can be
scanned in 9 s. The fast examination in combination with very low dose protocols
provides an excellent basis for preventive CT diagnosis with patient comfort and
safety.

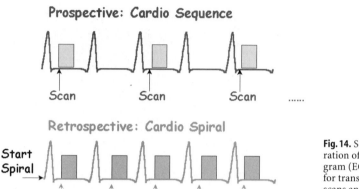

Fig. 14. Schematic illustration of electrocardiogram (ECG) triggering for transaxial multislice scans and of ECG gating for spiral multislice scans

Cardiac CT Imaging

In order to approach imaging of the heart, all of the previous elements are needed: volume coverage, breath hold scanning, and isotropic resolution. In addition, the best temporal resolution and synchronization of the data acquisition to the heart motion are essential elements. [5, 9]. Based on the 0.5-s full rotation, dedicated spiral algorithms presently provide 125 ms (60 ms as a limit) temporal resolution and are optimized with respect to volume coverage [5].

There are two methods for this synchronization: prospective ECG triggering of sequential scans and retrospective ECG gating of spiral scans [9]. Both methods are graphically sketched in Figure 14. Correspondingly, there are two cardiac CT protocols: multislice sequential scanning with the primary application to image and to quantify coronary calcifications [10] and multislice spiral scanning to access the morphology of the heart and of the coronaries [11].

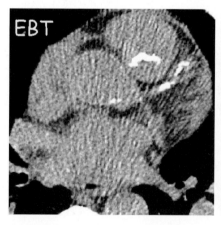
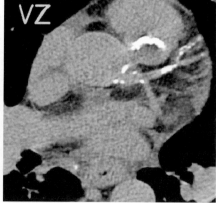

Fig. 15. Detection of coronary calcifications with electron beam computed tomography (EBCT) and multislice CT (SOMATOM Volume Zoom) in an obese patient

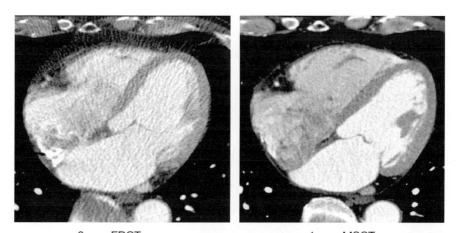

3 mm EBCT   1 mm MSCT

Fig. 16. Superior delineation of cardiac morphology with narrow collimation

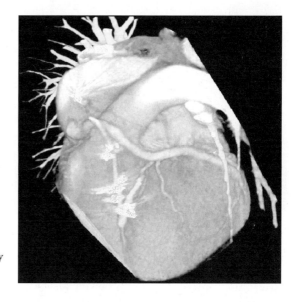

Fig. 17. Follow-up of bypass patency
with multislice computed tomography

Imaging of coronary calcifications has, for a long time, been the exclusive domain of EBCT. From the clinical studies available so far, it appears that ECG-guided multislice scanning is competitive with certain advantages (Fig. 15) in terms of the signal to noise (S/N) ratio and the reproducibility [12].

Similar to the non-cardiac applications, the ECG-guided spiral acquisition opens up a rich field of cardiac applications by acquiring continuous volume data sets close to isotropic resolution. The proper adaptation of the table feed to the heart rate of the patient is a prerequisite for the guarantee of gapless volume imaging [5]. In this respect, the free and continuous pitch selection is essential for efficient scanning at the lowest dose.

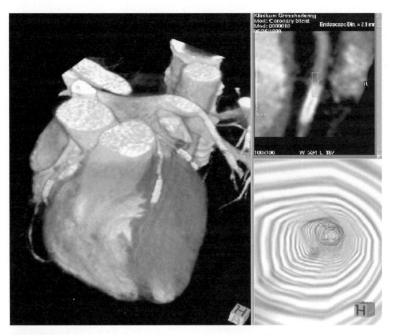

Fig. 18. Patency of stents with multislice computed tomography – endoluminal view in an endoscopic mode

High axial resolution with 4 x 1-mm collimation is the key to achieve excellent delineation of the small, anatomical structures (Fig. 16). Again, volumetric viewing and diagnosis in a volumetric mode are prerequisites for handling such high-quality 3D data sets (Fig. 2). The clinical capabilities of the technique are several fold [9, 11, 13, 14], such as follow-up after surgery or stent placement. The issues are patency of bypasses or stents. Endoscopic views are particularly helpful for evaluating the patency of stents (Fig. 17 and Fig. 18).

From an imaging standpoint, the detection of calcified plaques represents a high contrast situation. Given the proven low contrast resolution of the SOMA-TOM Volume Zoom, it is not surprising that also soft non-calcified plaques can be detected and visualized using MSCT. Figure 19 shows a representative example with corresponding stenoses in a 3D-rendered view. The correlation of the CT findings with the gold standards is an ongoing research activity, including correlation with angiography for stenoses and with intravascular ultrasound for soft plaque findings.

In order to optimize the methods for functional imaging and imaging at high heart rates, multislice spiral scanning offers another interesting and helpful feature for the maximization of the temporal resolution. The basic principle is to pick up the data either during one or two or four heart cycles and to fill the sinugram data correspondingly (Fig. 20). The effective temporal resolution can then be increased from 250 ms to 125 ms and to about 60 ms in the limit of a quadphasic algorithm.

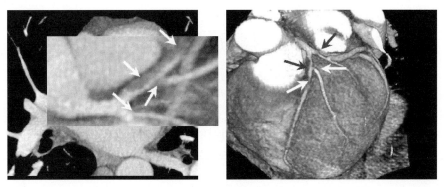

Fig. 19. Detection of soft, non-calcified plaques and their relation to stenoses in a three-dimensional-rendered view

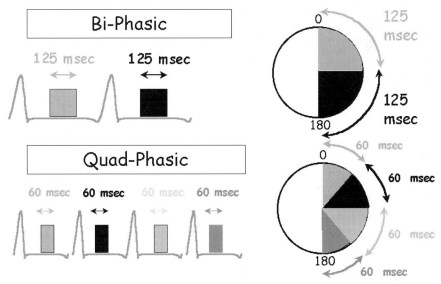

Fig. 20. The principle of multi-phasic acquisition and image reconstruction for optimized temporal resolution

One application of such optimized temporal resolution scans is the complete elimination of motion artifacts for coronary imaging at high heart rates. Figure 21 shows a comparison of images reconstructed with a monophasic and a biphasic algorithm, respectively, from the same data set. If functional information is aimed at, then such multi-phasic algorithms are of particular value. Figure 22 shows an example of imaging during systole with very pronounced improvements due to the improved elimination of the rapid motion during systole when multi-phasic algorithms are applied.

Summary and Outlook

Future extensions of multislice scanners with simultaneous read out of more slices will further extend the clinical uses which we saw developing over the last few years. It is expected that scanning with isotropic resolution will further evolve and will become standard. As a consequence, volumetric visualization and detection will to a large extent replace the traditional approach in a transaxial fashion. CT imaging of the coronaries and of the heart will be the method of choice for noninvasive imaging of the morphology in an easy to use, accurate, and reproducible manner. Multislice scanners will be the vehicle for screening applications.

High Heart Rate: ~95bpm

Diastole, Mono-Phasic   Diastole, Bi-Phasic

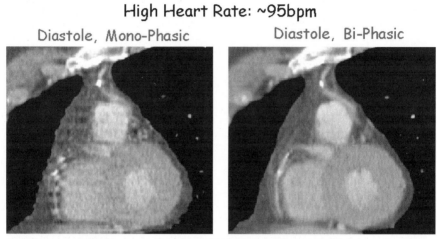

Fig. 21. Improvements of image quality using multi-phasic algorithms for high heart rates

High Heart Rate: ~95bpm

Systole, Mono-Phasic   Systole, Bi-Phasic

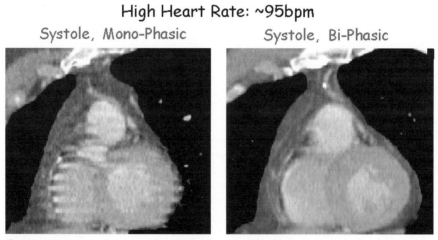

Fig. 22. Improvements of image quality using multi-phasic algorithms for imaging in systole

Obviously those future extensions of MSCT scanning require the close collaboration between clinicians and manufacturers in order to work out the proper clinical processes, dedicated applications, and the proper workflow for visualization and detection in order to handle the large amount of image data. It is easy to envision the creation of a CT "bodygram" in less than 20 s, consisting of 1-mm sections from the neck to the pubic symphysis. This will open new vistas for early disease detection and will change the way in which radiologists interact with the image data to improve patient care.

References

1. Kalender WA, Seissler W, Klotz E., Vock P (1990) Spiral volumetric CT with single-breath-hold technique, continuous transport and continuous scanner rotation. Radiology 176:181–183
2. Crawford CR, King KF (1990) Computed tomography scanning with simultaneous patient translation. Med Phys 17:967–982
3. Kalender WA (1995) Thin-section three-dimensional spiral CT: is isotropic imaging possible? Radiology 197:578–580
4. Klingenbeck-Regn K, Schaller S, Flohr T, Ohnesorge B, Kopp AF, Baum U (1999) Subsecond multislice computed tomography: basics and applications. Eur J Radiol 31:110–124
5. Ohnesorge B, Flohr T, Schaller S, Klingenbeck-Regn K, Becker C, Schöpf UJ, Brüning R, Reiser MF (1999) Technische Grundlagen und Anwendungen der Mehrschicht CT. Radiologe 39:923–931
6. Schaller S, Flohr T, Steffen P (1997) A new, efficient Fourier-reconstruction method for approximate image reconstruction in spiral cone-beam CT at small cone-angles. Proceedings of the SPIE international symposium on medical imaging 3032:213–224
7. Schaller S, Flohr T, Wolf H, Kalender WA (1999) Evaluation of a spiral reconstruction algorithm for multirow-CT. Radiology 209: 434
8. Schöpf UJ, Becker CR, Brüning R, Huber AM, Hong C (1999) Multidetector-array spiral CT imaging of focal and diffuse lung disease: thin-collimation data acquisition with reconstruction of contiguous and HRCT sections. Radiology 213(P): 258
9. Ohnesorge B, Flohr T, Becker C, Knez A, Kopp AF, Fukuda K, Reiser MF (2000) Herzbildgebung mit schneller, retrospektiv EKG-synchronisierter Mehrschichtspiral-CT. Radiologe 40:111–117
10. Becker CR, Knez A, Ohnesorge B, Flohr T, Schoepf UJ, Reiser M (1999) Detection and quantification of coronary artery calcifications with prospectively ECG triggered multirow conventional CT and electron beam computed tomography: comparison of different methods for quantification of coronary artery calcifications. Radiology 213(P): 351
11. Kopp AF, Ohnesorge B, Flohr T, Georg C, Schröder S, Küttner A, Martensen J, Claussen CD (2000) Multidetektor CT des Herzens: Erste klinische Anwendung einer retrospektiv EKG-gesteuerten Spirale mit optimierter zeitlicher und örtlicher Auflösung zur Darstellung der Herzkranzgefäße. Fortschr. Röntgenstr. 172:1–7
12. Ohnesorge B, Flohr T, Becker CR, Kopp AF, Knez A (1999) Comparison of EBCT and ECG-gated multislice spiral CT: a study of 3D Ca-scoring with phantom and patient data. Radiology 213(P): 402
13. Kopp AF, Georg C, Schröder S, Claussen CD (2000) CT-Angiographie der Herzkranzgefäße bei koronarer 3-Gefäß-Erkrankung. Fortschr. Röntgenstr. 172: 3–4
14. Kopp AF, Ohnesorge B, Flohr T, Schroeder S, Claussen CD (1999) Multidetector-row CT for the noninvasive detection of high-grade coronary artery stenoses and occlusions: first results. Radiology 213(P): 435

What is Changed in Contrast Medium Injection when Using High-Resolution Multislice Computed Tomography?

ROBERTO PASSARIELLO, CARLO CATALANO, FEDERICA PEDICONI,
ROBERTO BRILLO

In the past years, we have assisted with several technical developments which have totally changed the performances of computed tomography (CT) equipment. Starting from the early 1970s, the scan time was several minutes, the reconstruction time was almost 1 min, the minimum slice thickness was more than 1 cm, the matrix was limited, and the contrast resolution was poor. Now, in the late 1990s and the year 2000, there have been dramatic improvements in terms of speed of acquisition and reconstruction with a reduction of slice thickness to less than 1 mm and a significant increase of spatial resolution. These technical improvements also meant the possibility to perform new types of studies with CT previously not possible, such as, high resolution, dynamic evaluation of parenchymal organs and lesions, and non-invasive angiographies.

The faster acquisition has also determined an increase in velocity of contrast media (c.m.) administration: drip infusion has been substituted by bolus injection with power injectors [1]. At the same time, contrast agents had to be injected at faster flow rates and, most importantly, the timing between c.m. administration and scanning had to be calculated. The experience of several years has shown that the time arrival of the c.m. is strictly related to the heart rate of the patient and to the patient's cardiac output. Already with the latest sequential scanners, the circulation time and as a consequence the delay time, could be grossly calculated knowing the heart rate of the patient [2].

After the introduction of spiral CT, the mode of c.m. administration has again changed. It is evident that the best contrast enhancement is obtained when the maximum concentration of iodine in the scanned volume is reached during the effective acquisition temporal window. To reach the best contrast enhancement, several different modes of injection have been proposed. These are either uniphasic or biphasic [3]. Nevertheless, none of them has provided a prolonged optimal vascular enhancement, to obtain which a mode of injection tailored for each patient was needed, as shown by Fleischmann et al. [4]. Although the customized administration of contrast agent appears the most efficacious, it is rarely utilized in the clinical practice, being complicated and making the examination more prolonged. In multislice spiral CT, the temporal window for c.m. administration has been further reduced by about eight times relative to single-slice spiral CT, with 1 s gantry rotation time.

The contrast enhancement in all CT examinations, but significantly more in spiral CT, depends upon several factors: the amount of contrast agent, the injection flow rate, the synchronization with scanning, the type of vascularization of organs and lesions, the contrast to noise ratio, and finally, the type of contrast medium and its main features (osmolarity, viscosity, vascular persistence, and iodine concentration).

The amount of c.m. administered has a limited and relative significance in arterial enhancement. The enhancement in the venous and parenchymatous phases is determined by the amount of c.m. administered. Therefore, if a multislice CT arterial study has to be performed, there is no need to administer large amounts of c.m.; the overall quantity can be easily calculated according to the patient circulation time and imaging window. If a CT study in a venous-delayed phase must be performed, larger quantities of c.m. must be injected to obtain a sufficient venous enhancement in order also to avoid and limit the excessive dilution of the contrast agent.

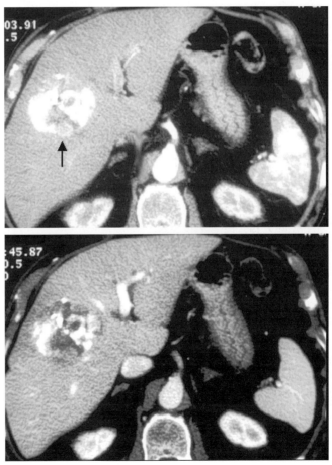

Fig. 1. HCC at the multislice computed tomography in the early arterial phase shows, in the posterior part of a previously treated HCC, a nodular recurrency (*arrow*), which is fainted in the portal venous vein

The correct injection flow rate is crucial to obtain a good arterial enhancement but has a limited importance for what regards the paranchymatous and venous enhancement. Nevertheless, in consideration of the limited acquisition temporal window, a compromise has to be made between the amount of contrast material (c.m.) administered and the flow rate. Therefore, a high flow rate has to be utilized, particularly when a fast scanning protocol (4 x 5-mm collimation thickness) is applied [5].

In order to obtain an excellent arterial enhancement, the c.m. administration has to be correctly synchronized with scanning (Fig. 1); in consideration of the short scanning time, the possibility of timing errors is significantly higher than with single-slice spiral CT. The same method for determination of the delay time of single-slice spiral CT can be applied to multislice spiral CT (although they appear more useful in the latter) not only in angiographic studies but also in the assessment of parenchymal organs. A correct synchronization is crucial not only for lesion detection but also for characterization. In fact, the type of vascularization can be well demonstrated, particularly if correct timing is utilized (Fig. 2).

The type of c.m. utilized appears also important in multislice spiral CT. The osmolarity and viscosity of c.m. have a limited significance on arterial, venous, and parenchymatous enhancement, although they may determine variations in flow rate. Although there have been several attempts to prepare contrast agents with a prolonged vascular persistence, similar to intravascular c.m. for magnetic resonance imaging (MRI), the increased scanning speed reduces the need to increase intravascular persistence. A c.m. feature that is gaining an increased

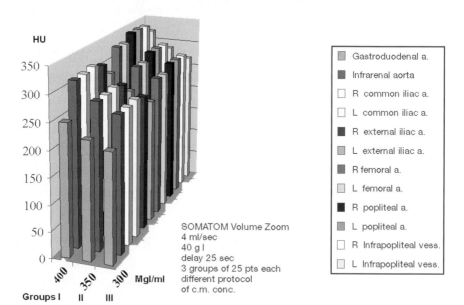

Fig. 2. Peripheral artery enhancement study using different contrast media concentration: in all of the arterial segments examined, it is possible to visualize an increase of enhancement using a higher concentration of iodine

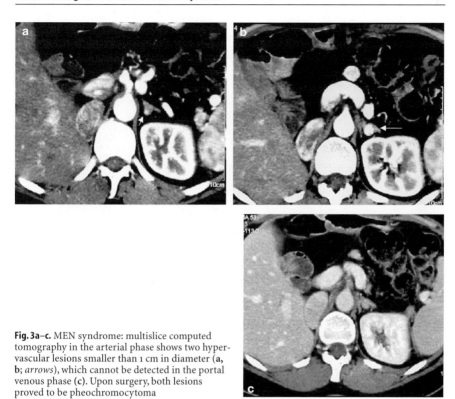

Fig. 3a–c. MEN syndrome: multislice computed tomography in the arterial phase shows two hypervascular lesions smaller than 1 cm in diameter (**a, b**; *arrows*), which cannot be detected in the portal venous phase (**c**). Upon surgery, both lesions proved to be pheochromocytoma

importance in multislice spiral CT is the iodine concentration. In fact, the limited temporal window may be overcome by a high iodine concentration, particularly in the arterial phase of the study.

In our institution, we performed a study comparison of CT angiography (CTA). We used three contrast agents with different iodine concentrations (400 mgI/ml, 350 mgI/ml, and 300 mgI/ml) and administered a standard dose of iodine (40 g/examination) corresponding to 100 ml of 400 mgI/ml, 113 ml of 350 mgI/ml, and 133 ml of 300 mgI/ml. Density values were calculated using standard ROIs in several arterial segments from the aorta to the distal trifurcation vessels. Although the same amount of iodine was utilized, there was a significant increase of attenuation values in the arteries proportional to the concentration of I/ml. The increase of attenuation values (but overall of the distal vessels' visibility and enhancement) in the visual analysis has been significant using a c.m. with 400 mgI/ml (Fig. 3). All manufacturers of c.m. are now evaluating the possibility of developing a c.m. with even higher concentration, which may be particularly useful in cases of very short scanning time during which a high concentration of iodine must be rapidly reached. An important aspect in multislice spiral CT is the flow rate to be utilized. In general, we may say that it depends on the scanned volume and scanning time. Therefore, we have to make a distinction between examinations of single organs with the purpose of performing tissue characte-

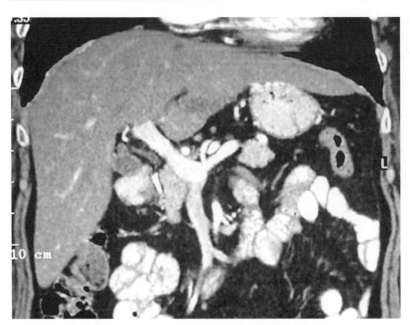

Fig. 4. The thin slice acquisition with a flow rate of 3 ml/s provides an excellent portal venous opacification

rization, functional studies, and exams of large volumes, particularly of vascular structures using a thin-slice collimation. In the first case, a higher flow rate (5–6 ml/s) has to be utilized in order to administer during the short scanning time a consistent amount of c.m. In case of prolonged acquisition, the flow rate can be reduced (3–4 ml/s) without affecting the overall amount administered (Fig. 4).

CT Angiography (CTA)

In multislice spiral CTA, the amount of contrast agent may vary according to the scanning volume and time. If a small volume (intracranial circulation, carotid arteries) is studied, a limited amount of c.m. can be utilized and injected at a high flow rate. The same injection protocol can be applied also when assessing the pulmonary vasculature in cases of suspected pulmonary embolism [6]. In all of these examples, multislice spiral CT allows a reduction of the overall amount of IV c.m. of at least 35% but even greater in most cases. When large volumes must be scanned, the amount of IV c.m. necessarily is increased, although still limited relative to single-slice spiral CT.

Particularly when a limited volume is studied and the scanning time is short, it is advisable to avoid too early or delayed studies, to perform a test bolus sequence, or to find a method for determination of bolus arrival. By performing a test bolus, the possibility of errors is limited to a small percentage.

Body CT

In body CT, the amount of c.m. relative to single-slice spiral CT can be reduced if a limited volume is scanned. The flow velocity is mainly determined by the slice thickness and a consequence of the scanning time. If an upper abdomen or a thorax study has to be performed using a 5 mm collimation, the flow rate must be high (4–6 ml/s) in order to administer an adequate amount of iodinated contrast agent in a short time. If the acquisition is more prolonged, for instance in the case of thin-slice collimation, the contrast agent can be injected at a slower rate (3 ml/s). Therefore, the flow rate and, as a consequence, the volume injected, must be modified according to the type of study to be performed and the scanning time. In conclusion, after the introduction of multislice spiral CT, one of the main problems to be solved, is the modality of c.m. administration [7]. The overall quantity, flow rate, and type of c.m. to be utilized still need to be determined. With regard to the c.m. amount, it seems from this early experience that significantly reduced doses can be utilized relative to single-slice spiral CT, particularly for what concerns CTA examinations. Customized protocols may be useful for obtaining a constant and prolonged vascular enhancement, although they may require complicated calculations not strictly necessary. The technique of multi-slice spiral CT is brand new and experimental studies are needed also to determine the best c.m. to be injected and the modality of administration.

References

1. R. Passariello (1985) Angio-CT techniques. Eur J Radiol 5:193–198
2. R.Passariello et al. (1980) Automatic contrast medium injector for computer tomography. J Comput Assist Tomogr, 4:278–279
3. Heiken et al.(1993) Dynamic contrast-enhanced CT of the liver: comparison of contrast medium injection rates and uniphasic and biphasic injection protocols. Radiology 187:327–331
4. Fleischmann et al. (1999) Mathematical analysis of arterial enhancement and optimization of bolus geometry for CT angiography using the discrete Fourier transform. J Comput Assist Tomogr 23:474–484
5. Blomley et al. (1997) Bolus dynamics: theoretical and experimental aspects. Br J Radiol 70:351–359
6. Brink et al. (1997) Depiction of pulmonary emboli with spiral CT: optimization of display window settings in a porcine model. Radiology 204:703–708
7. Luboldt et al. (1999) Effective contrast use in CT angiography and dual-phase hepatic CT performed with a subsecond scanner. Invest Radiol 26:751–760

Computer Modeling Approach to Contrast Medium Administration and Scan Timing for Multislice Computed Tomography

Kyongtae T. Bae, Jay P. Heiken

Rationale for Computer Modeling of Contrast Enhancement

Proper scan timing after contrast medium administration has always been important for computed tomography (CT). With the introduction of multislice CT, the need for proper scan timing has become even more critical because of the very short acquisition time for multislice examinations. Studies that took 20–30 s to acquire with single slice CT now can be acquired in less than 10 s. If scan timing is not optimized, the appropriate phase of contrast medium enhancement can be missed. Computer modeling can serve as the basis for a completely automated CT scanning optimization system for multislice examinations when it is integrated with a low-dose prescanning technique for contrast medium bolus monitoring.

Our current understanding of intravenous (IV) contrast medium enhancement is complicated by multiple interacting factors: contrast medium type, contrast medium volume and concentration, injection technique, catheter size and site, imaging technique, patient characteristics, and tissue characteristics. The variables that cannot be controlled are those related to the patient (i.e., age gender, weight, height, cardiovascular status, and the presence of other diseases).

The large body of physiologic data available for the human cardiovascular system allows us to estimate the propagation and distribution of contrast medium throughout the human body. When we consider contrast medium as a pharmaceutical injected intravenously, its concentration can be predicted by using mathematical techniques developed in pharmacokinetics [1]. The distribution of contrast medium in an organ depends on the organ's perfusion rate, tissue volume, tissue composition, and permeabilities throughout the organ microvasculature and cellular interfaces. A whole-body system can be modeled by applying mass balances for each organ and tissue and then by integrating organs with appropriate perfusion distributions. Thus, organ-specific contrast medium enhancement can be computed for given input parameters. We have developed such a model [2].

Cardiovascular System

A simplified human cardiovascular system consists of the heart, vascular networks, and key organs (such as the lungs, the visceral organs, the trunk, and the

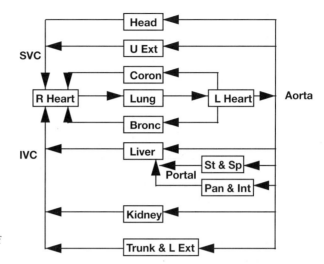

Fig. 1. Schematic diagram of circulation system

extremities) that serve as reservoirs (Fig. 1). To describe a standard model of the cardiovascular system, we obtained from the physiology literature the average blood volume and cardiac output values for a typical 70-kg adult. We then adjusted the values according to the input patient's gender, weight, and height by using standard nomograms incorporated into our computer model.

Distribution of Body Fluid

Since contrast medium is not confined within the vascular space but diffuses passively across the capillary membrane into the extravascular space, its distribution is closely related to that of total body fluid, which is approximately 57% of total body weight. We divided total body fluid into two major compartments: intracellular fluid (ICF) and extracellular fluid (ECF). The ECF was further divided into several smaller compartments, the largest of which is interstitial fluid. The ECF volume used in our model was based on the volume of distribution of iohexol, 0.27 l/kg [3]. The detailed distribution of fluid in a local organ was estimated from the standard mass of the organ and its fluid content.

Modeling of a Blood Vessel and the Heart

Local structures were modeled mathematically to describe the distribution and dispersion of intravascularly administered iodinated contrast medium within local regions. Blood vessels were modeled as rigid structures with a well-mixed pool of blood and contrast medium. A well-mixed compartment contains a constant volume with a single inlet flow and a single outlet flow. The input and output flow rates are the same. Since we assume the compartment is well-mixed, the concentration within the compartment is the same as that of the output. A mass balance on the concentration is described by the Fick principle. For a given volume, flow rate, and input concentration, we can estimate the output concentration by solving the differential equation described by the Fick principle.

Modeling an Organ

Modeling an organ requires consideration of transcapillary exchange of contrast medium between the vascular and interstitial spaces. We divided each organ into three well-described spaces: the capillary or intravascular space; the extravascular, extracellular space; and the intracellular space. Diffusion through membranes permits exchange of substances among the spaces within an organ. However, because iodinated contrast medium does not penetrate the cells, we considered only the intravascular and extracellular compartments and ignored the intracellular compartment. Transcapillary exchange of substances between the intravascular and extracellular compartments can be described by the Fick law of diffusion. Two additional governing differential equations were applied to each organ, one for the intravascular space and the other for the extracellular space.

Modeling of a Global Circulation System

A global model, described using 104 ordinary differential equations, was formed by integrating regional circulation parameters with the models of local regions. The equations were solved with a numeric integration program (Runge-Kutta method [4]). To adjust the model size for patient variation, regression formulas were used to predict blood volume and cardiac output for a given patient's gender, weight, and height.

Relationship between Iodine Concentration and CT Enhancement

To understand the relationship between iodine concentration and CT enhancement, we performed a simple experiment which demonstrated that an increase in concentration of 1 mg of iodine per milliliter yields approximately 25 HU of contrast enhancement (Fig. 2).

Completed Model

The model described above can be run on a personal computer and takes less than 1 s to compute. The curve of contrast medium concentration over time can be calculated for each region by solving differential equations of the global model for a given contrast medium injection protocol and a patient of specific weight, height, and gender.

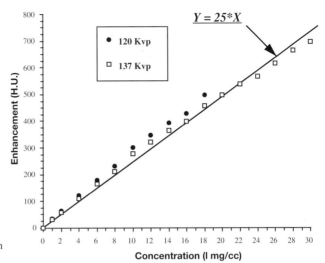

Fig. 2. The relationship between iodine concentration and CT enhancement for two different kVp settings. Assuming a linear relationship, an increase in concentration by 1 mgI/ml yields an increase in CT attenuation by approximately 25 H.U.

Model Validation

Pooled Data

Aortic and hepatic CT contrast medium enhancement curves were simulated for three contrast medium injection protocols and were compared with the mean enhancement curves from three groups of 25–28 patients receiving the same injection protocols. The simulation of CT contrast medium enhancement for each protocol was based on a hypothetical patient whose weight matched the average weight in each experimental protocol group. The mean percent difference in maximum enhancement was 7.4% for the aortic curves and 4.8% for the hepatic curves. The curves also were nearly identical in variation over time.

Individual Data

Patients (240) referred for abdominal CT were randomized into four protocol groups in which the injection rates and concentrations and volumes of contrast medium were varied. The aortic and hepatic contrast enhancement curves of these patients were measured and compared with the enhancement curves predicted by the computer program. The mean percent difference in maximum enhancement between the empiric and simulated curves was 5.3% for the aorta and 6% for the liver.

Practical Application

Despite numerous clinical studies of IV contrast medium enhancement techniques for body CT, our daily practice of injecting contrast medium, in many respects, is still based on our subjective experience and intuition rather than on

rigorous quantitative analysis of the mechanism of contrast medium enhancement. Our computer model of the human cardiovascular system has many potential clinical applications. It can predict organ-specific contrast enhancement in a
patient with a specific body habitus subjected to different contrast medium
injection protocols. In so doing, it can help determine the adequacy of an injection protocol to achieve a desired level of enhancement in an organ of interest
and thus can be useful in optimizing contrast medium usage.

The model also has the potential to be useful in optimizing scanning timing
for both single- and dual-phase multislice CT examinations when it is integrated
with a low-dose prescanning technique for contrast medium bolus monitoring.
Our model is based on the presumption of normal cardiac output, and thus may
not accurately predict the timing of contrast medium enhancement when the
cardiac output of a patient deviates greatly from the predicted normal value. A
method of adjusting scanning timing based on the cardiac variability of an
individual patient may be to use the aortic enhancement pattern obtained from
bolus-tracking techniques with low X-ray dose monitoring CT scans. The aortic
enhancement pattern reflects the patient's cardiac output status and can be
integrated with the model to modify the prediction accounting for cardiac output
variability.

Another way in which the computer model can be used is to solve the inverse
problem, i.e., to predict an input function for a given output contrast enhancement profile. Thus, if we know the shape we would like the aortic enhancement

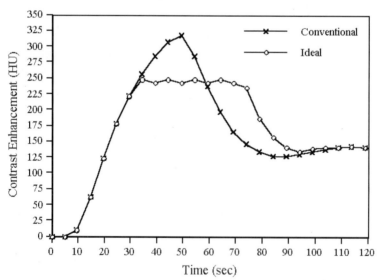

Fig. 3. A typical and a desired contrast medium enhancement curve. A typical aortic enhancement
curve was simulated on a hypothetical adult male with a fixed height (173 cm) and body weight
(68 kg), subject to injection of 160 ml of 320 mgI/ml contrast agent at 4 ml/s. This shows a steadily
rising vascular contrast enhancement profile with a single peak of enhancement, resulting in non-
uniform enhancement during image acquisition. Uniform vascular enhancement through the entire
period of image acquisition is highly desirable for efficient use of contrast medium and for image
processing and display

curve to have, we can use the model to design an injection technique that would result in the desired enhancement curve (Fig. 3). We have used this method to design a novel, multi-phasic contrast injection method that generates prolonged uniform vascular enhancement for CT angiography (CTA) [5].

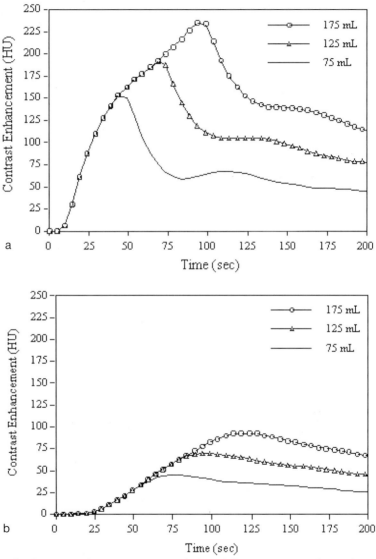

Fig. 4a, b. Simulated contrast enhancement curves with three different contrast medium volumes. Simulated enhancement curves of the aorta (**a**) and liver (**b**) based on a hypothetical adult male with a fixed height (173 cm) and body weight (68 kg), subject to injection of 75, 125, and 175 ml of 320 mgI/ml contrast agent at 2 ml/s. The time to peak enhancement and the magnitude of the peak enhancement increases with increasing contrast medium volume

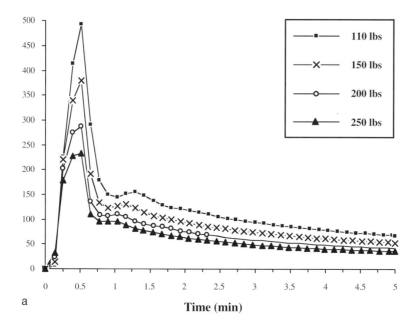

a

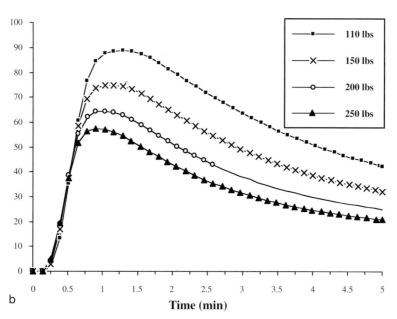

b

Fig. 5a, b. Simulated contrast enhancement curves with four different body weights. Simulated enhancement curves of the aorta **(a)** and liver **(b)** based on a hypothetical adult male with a fixed height (173 cm) and varying body weight (50, 73, 91, 118 kg), subject to injection of 125 ml of 320 mgI/ml contrast agent at 5 ml/s. The magnitude of contrast enhancement is inversely proportional to the body weight

Finally, this model may be useful in improving our understanding of the effects of various physiologic and pharmacokinetic parameters on CT contrast medium enhancement, such as contrast medium volume (Fig. 4), body weight (Fig. 5), and cardiac output (Fig. 6). Such improved understanding of the mechanisms underlying contrast medium enhancement may enable us to further optimize our contrast medium injection techniques for patients with various pathologic conditions.

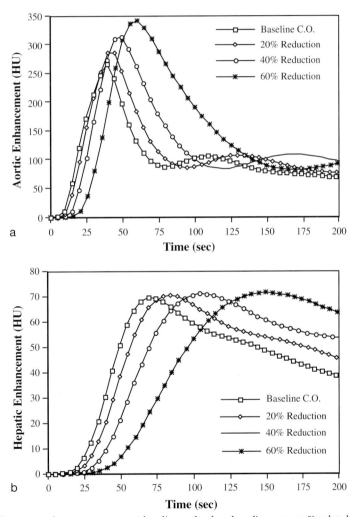

Fig. 6a, b. Simulated contrast enhancement curves at baseline and reduced cardiac outputs. Simulated enhancement curves of the aorta (**a**) and liver (**b**) based on a hypothetical adult male with a fixed height (173 cm) and body weight (68 kg), subject to injection of 120 ml of 320 mgI/ml contrast agent at 4 ml/s. A set of aortic and hepatic contrast enhancement curves were generated from the model by reducing the baseline (normal) cardiac output, i.e., 6500 ml/min by 20, 40, and 60%

References

1. Gerlowski L, Jain R (1983) Physiologically based pharmacokinetic modeling: principles and applications. J Pharm Sci 72:1103–1127
2. Bae KT, Heiken JP, Brink JA (1998) Aortic and hepatic contrast medium enhancement at CT: part I. Prediction with a computer model. Radiology 207:647–655
3. Olsson B, Aulie A, Sveen K, Andrew E (1983) Human pharmacokinetics of iohexol: a new nonionic contrast medium. Invest Radiol 18:177–182
4. Press WH, Flannery BP, Teukolsky SA, Vetterling WT (1986) Numerical recipes. Cambridge University Press, Cambridge
5. Bae KT, Tran HQ, Heiken JP (2000) Multiphasic contrast injection method to generate uniform prolonged vascular enhancement: pharmacokinetic analysis and Experimental porcine model. Radiology 216:872–880

Three-Dimensional Imaging and Virtual Reality Applications of Multislice Computed Tomography

SIMON WILDERMUTH, NINOSLAV TEODOROVIC, PAUL R. HILFIKER, BORUT MARINCEK

Introduction

A few years ago, a discussion of three-dimensional (3D) and virtual reality imaging might have been overly futuristic and perhaps of marginal interest to those in clinical practice. However, the rapid rise of techniques, such as computed tomography angiography (CTA) and magnetic resonance angiography (MRA) and the development of multislice CT (MSCT) with data files that now reach a thousand slices per data set, demand 3D solutions.

This chapter will emphasize the applications of 3D imaging that are being used with MSCT, particularly those that emphasize surface and volume rendering (VR). These applications are examples of the most important aspects of 3D imaging. In addition, this chapter will cover virtual reality applications of MSCT, such as virtual endoscopy (VE) and surgical planning.

MSCT can capture four slices of data with a single rotation of the gantry. This allows for a dramatic increase in speed and a dramatic increase in anatomic coverage with very little penalty [1] and has driven 3D imaging and virtual reality intensively. This development has eliminated misregistration artifacts and respiratory artifacts, thereby achieving true volumetric imaging [2, 3]. Imaging will move from the flat picture of a 2D display to the perspective revealed by a 3D display. This is an imaging renaissance. Anatomic relationships that could not be fully appreciated before are being revealed through advanced data sets. Numerous applications of 3D imaging have clinical relevance. Looking at a tumor's response to therapy in terms of tumor volumetrics performed in 3D imaging would be more objective and more statistically accurate [4, 5]. 3D imaging could immensely enhance much of the work being performed with 2D imaging.

MS scanners can now perform peripheral vascular CT, allowing clinicians to scan from the diaphragm to the toes in a minute. The problem is that the scan produces a thousand images, a number that does not lend itself to traditional 2D display, let alone filming. These images must be viewed in 3D [6]. Coronal multiplanar reconstruction (MPR), automated surface rendering or VR can be very helpful for displaying the entire anatomy. The transition from step and shoot dynamic CT to spiral CT was revolutionary. There are many clinical applications that can now be done with breath-held volume imaging data sets, but the revolution due to the new hardware was only realized when the software for CTA was developed. The same is somewhat true with MSCT. Therefore, although MSCT is faster and extends the ability to perform CTA, for example, its full impact will not be felt until software innovation, such as real-time 3D has been developed. Spiral and MSCT scanning are critically important hardware developments in terms of speed of acquisition, but in order to use these in the clinical practice, the software to enable better 3D and CTA imaging must be available. Another importance is the interactivity of the 3D software. Although at many times data sets still must be off-loaded to specific work stations, vendors understand that this information must be available in real time and, that in the near future, the images must pop out of the machine.

The development of MSCT, achieving true volumetric imaging, also has an enormous impact in medical virtual reality applications. Surgical simulation has many applications in medical education, surgical training, surgical planning, and intra-operative assistance. However, extending current surface-based computer graphics methods to model phenomena, such as the deformation, cutting, tearing, or repairing of soft tissues, poses significant challenges for real-time interactions. The use of volumetric methods for modeling complex anatomy and tissue interactions becomes close to reality using high-resolution MSCT data sets. New techniques are introduced that use volumetric methods for modeling soft-tissue deformation and tissue cutting at interactive rates, visual feedback via real-time VR and polygon rendering and haptic feedback provided by a force-feedback device.

Techniques

Multi-planar Reconstruction

The 3D nature of volume images allows for simple and efficient computation of images that lie along the non-acquired orthogonal orientations of the volume [7]. This is accomplished by readdressing the order of voxels in the volume image, which can be done interactively when the volume image is entirely stored in the memory of a computer. It is a very fast and interactive algorithm, suitable to represent several arbitrary planes at once. Implementations of MPR techniques on modern computers allow for an interactive generation and display of these images in real time on multi-panel displays.

From the early days of CT, MPR is being used as a tool to provide arbitrary planes from transaxial slices. MPR, however, is not considered to be a true 3D representation, and the image quality is limited by the z-resolution of the CT data set. Therefore, MPRs have not been used much in conventional CT since spatial resolution along the z-axis used to be poor and stair-step artifacts were common. With the advent of MSCT with the possibility of isotropic data sets, stair-step artifacts can be eliminated, but image quality still depends on acquisition parameters. Using thin collimation, excellent results are obtained (Fig. 1). Generally, MPRs are helpful whenever pathology cannot be accurately assessed on axial images alone. Most situations involve pathologic interfaces that are oriented parallel to the axial plane or structures that cannot be displayed in their entirety since they run through a number of slices. In these cases, problem-oriented imaging planes can be generated using MPR. Newer 3D visualization techniques

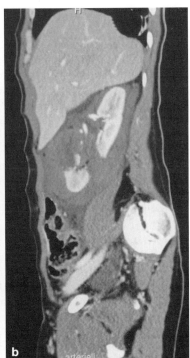

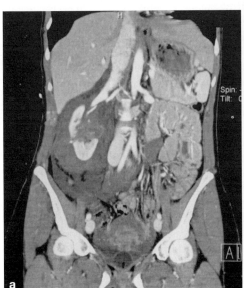

Fig. 1a, b. The ability of computed tomography (CT) to recon on the fly. This emergency CT study shows multiple views of an abdominal trauma case with retroperitoneal bleeding caused by a ruptured kidney. Excellent multi-planar reconstruction images allow radiologists and surgeons to make a correct diagnosis and overview within a few seconds and enable a very fast workflow in the emergency room. However, many more slices were generated with MSCT than older techniques used previously

could take over this role. However, MPR is still the fastest reconstruction method and available almost everywhere where CT images are acquired.

For accurate diagnosis and surgical planning on most complex calcaneal fractures, conventional CT images were obtained at least in two different planes. Today, multiple high quality MPR, based on one MSCT data set with nearly isotropic resolution, can substitute for the extra images that used to be obtained with standard CT to yield axial and coronal views of the fracture lines and the various calcaneal joints. MPRs also serve as an important communication tool with the referring physicians and play a major role in orthopedic and trauma therapy planning.

Surface Rendering (Shaded Surface Display)

The "Marching Cubes" algorithm must be considered the hallmark of surface rendering. It is a table-based surface-fitting algorithm which generates triangle-based isosurfaces within 3D space [8]. Prior to applying the algorithm, the user specifies a threshold value. This specification has vast ramifications regarding the quality and accuracy of the object depiction. The threshold needs to be adapted to the individual application under consideration. As a guideline, the threshold should be chosen close to the center of the signal difference between the brightest pixel found within the object of interest and the signal in the surrounding structures. Once the threshold has been determined, the surface rendering algorithm loops on each successive group of four adjacent data slices. The slices are read into memory and each cell is scanned to determine whether its corner values straddle the threshold value. Non-straddling cells are discarded. Cells that do straddle the threshold are examined more closely. The eight corners of the cube are valued "1" if their signal exceeds the threshold and "0" if it does not. They form an eight-bit byte, which is treated as an index in a precomputed edge intersection table. The edge intersection lookup function returns 12 booleans, indicating which of the 12 edges of the cell are intersected by the isosurface. Interpolation is used to locate the edge intersected by the isosurface. If it is assumed that each edge can be intersected only once, four triangles are sufficient to depict the path of the isosurface through the cell. Groups of three cell edge intersection points are grouped to form triangles.

Surface rendering, also called shaded surface display (SSD), was mainly used to communicate findings to the referring physicians during the last decade. Using larger data sets performing MSCT, this visualization role will be overtaken by newer VR techniques. However, surface rendering still provides the basis for the planning of complex surgical procedures. While surface rendering images are very intuitive, they are also prone to artifacts since image quality is strongly dependent on the chosen threshold range for the definition of the displayed 3D object.

When performing polygon-based 3D models, it has to be stated that all information is already present on the 2D images and that SSD represent processed displays of the same information. Many radiologists, therefore, consider 3D displays as redundant. However, there are many applications in which radiology truly benefits from SSD. These include all procedures for surgical planning and 3D renderings of complex acetabular fractures, facial fractures, orthopedic deformities, CTA of the thoracic aorta, and preoperative planning for interventional endovascular procedures. The classification of acetabular fractures is markedly simplified with 3D reconstructions [9, 10]. Patients requiring complex surgical procedures showed the highest benefit, with significantly reduced operation time [11]. Complex procedures in craniofacial surgery also benefited from surface rendering for many years, where surgical planning was based either on SSD alone or on stereolitographic 3D models [12, 13].

In MSCTA, the SSD are still useful for visualization of complex anatomic situations, such as pathology of the thoracic and abdominal aorta [14] (Fig. 2). Its role for visualization of small aortic side branches is limited, where maximum intensity projections (MIP) and VR techniques are generally superior. The main advantage of MIP and VR over SSD is the preservation of density information. The wall calcifications and the contrasted vascular lumen can be differentiated. MIP images are not threshold-dependent, but a single MIP does not provide 3D

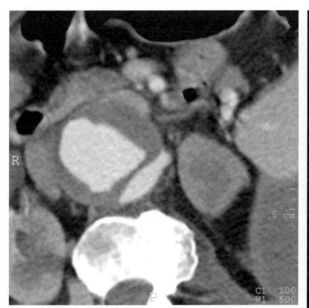
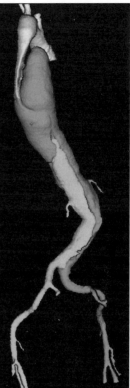

Fig. 2. Multislice computed tomography (MSCT) allows the clinician to scan from the aortic arch to the iliac arteries in a matter of seconds and to get excellent spatial resolution. If the functional information that magnetic resonance imaging (MRI) beautifully provides is not needed, MSCT has a lot to offer in terms of spatial resolution. This patient has a dissection in the thoracic and abdominal aorta. Shaded surface display allows an excellent differentiation between the luminas in this case

information. Therefore, foreground and background cannot be differentiated. In surgical planning for extensive aneurysms or dissections, the spatial relationship between pathologic areas and branching vessels is demonstrated to the best advantage. For imaging of aortic stents, SSD are a quick method to display the basic anatomy, screen for endograft leakages, and evaluate the ideal localization of the stent placement.

Volume Rendering

Volume rendering (VR) is the representation, visualization, and manipulation of objects represented as sampled data in three or more dimensions. VR differs from conventional 3D graphics in that traditional graphics represent object surfaces and boundaries using polygons or triangles [15]. VR displays visual images directly from volume data, enabling the viewer to fully reveal the internal structure of 3D data. Rather than editing a single scan, VR interpolates the entire data set. Speaking of MSCT and image postprocessing, VR is one of the most important software techniques. It will continue to aid in the display of this volumetric data well into the future. VR is interactive, and it allows quick scans through the large MSCT data sets and provides a comprehensive view of the anatomic situation, especially for those clinicians who are not familiar with reviewing cross-sectional images [16]. In addition, unlike other projection techniques, such as surface display and MIP, VR does not distort objects. With standard orthographic imaging, such as SSD or MIP, changing position can cause distortions in the image. With perspective VR, there is no distortion. Perspective VR requires a data set that permits 3D imaging, which basically means one with thin collimation. MSCT fulfills all these requirements and supplies isotropic data sets.

The rendering is performed using a software technique that assigns both opacity and color to each voxel in the data set. This VR engine can be implemented in either an image- or object order. The image order approach is generally referred to as 'ray-casting' [15]. It scans the display screen and, by casting a viewing ray, determines for each pixel which volume cells are affected by it. The opacities and shaded colors encountered along the ray are summed to determine the opacity and color of the corresponding pixel. The object order approach processes a list of volume cells based on their visibility order and determines for each volume cell which pixels are affected by it (Fig. 3). For the most part, the rendering process has been performed off line by a workstation that is either in a 3D lab or in a stand-alone facility adjacent to the CT suite. The near future will hopefully see the rendering process incorporated into the scan, meaning that VR displays will instantaneously emerge from a CT scanner.

Once the VR display has been compiled, the opacity can be suppressed in order to examine different tissues. If clinicians want to look at high attenuation structures, suppressing some of the low attenuation, the abdominal wall and the solid viscera can be subtracted away, leaving the skeletal structures. If they want to examine everything, then they can see a 3D image of the abdominal wall. If they wanted to examine something in between these two extremes, such as to

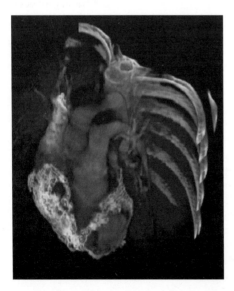

Fig. 3. Volume rendering of a case with extensive pericarditis constrictiva calcarea. Cardiac imaging is one of the last great frontiers for radiology, and it poses huge problems in terms of temporal and spatial resolution. There is great hope that very fast computed tomography imaging using multisclice technology may help in the evaluation of cardiac and coronary artery disease

suppress the subcutaneous fat and look at solid viscera, they have that option. VR provides great flexibility in terms of varying opacity curves. Lighting effects come into play as well; objects can be displayed differently depending on where a light source is shined into a data set, whether the interest lies in the skeletal structure or solid viscera. VR is the main 3D technique to display soft tissue structures even if no prior editing is employed. There are several potential advantages over SSD. However, VR plays a minor role in the field of surgical simulation. The main disadvantage of VR is still the large calculation effort that makes the procedure cumbersome to run on small workstations or personal computers.

Virtual Endoscopy

Virtual endoscopy (VE) describes a new method of diagnosis, using computer processing of 3D image data sets (such as from spiral or MSCT scans) to provide simulated visualizations of patient-specific organs similar or equivalent to those produced with standard endoscopic procedures [17, 18]. VE can be performed using surface rendering or VR based either on volumetric CT or MR data sets [19]. Thousands of endoscopic examinations are performed yearly. These procedures are invasive, often uncomfortable, and may cause serious side effects, such as perforation, infection, and hemorrhage. VE avoids these risks and, when used prior to a standard endoscopic exam, may minimize procedural difficulties, decreasing the morbidity rate. Additionally, VE allows for exploration of body regions that are inaccessible or incompatible with standard endoscopic procedures.

The recent availability of true isotropic data sets from MSCT examinations, coupled with the development of computer algorithms to accurately and rapidly render high-resolution images in 3D and perform fly-throughs provides a rich opportunity to take this new methodology from theory and preliminary studies to practice. Virtual visualizations of the trachea, esophagus, and colon have been compared to standard endoscopic views by endoscopists who judge them to be realistic and useful. Quantitative measurements of geometric and densitometric information obtained from the VE images have been carried out and compared with direct measures on the original data. These studies suggest that VE can provide accurate and reproducible visualizations and demonstrate significant promise for use in routine diagnostic screening. Small blood vessels and color of inflamed regions are often important diagnostic features that are not captured with MSCT imaging. Artificial texture mapping can be used to enhance realism in the computed endoscopic views, but this is not patient-specific and can be misleading. However, precise location, size, and shape of abnormal structures, such as lesions and masses can be accurately visualized with VE from any orientation, both within and outside of the region of interest. These capabilities are not possible with conventional endoscopy. And these can be obtained without inserting an uncomfortable probe into the body. This is the promise and rationale for VE as a screening procedure.

VE procedures performed with MSCT data sets have the potential to replace invasive procedures, such as colonoscopy or bronchoscopy. As examples, this

chapter will now describe in particular the potential application of virtual colonoscopy and virtual bronchoscopy. VE technologies can also be used in the bladder. Once the bladder is filled with air or regular iodinated contrast, a light source
can be directed into the area. Recent developments demonstrate the feasibility of
color mapping of bladder wall thickness, which differentiates both, normal, and
thickened urothelium [20].

Virtual Colonoscopy

Colorectal cancer is a high-profile clinical problem [21], but unlike many other
forms of cancer (lung cancer, carcinoma of the breast, and so forth), the cause of
this disease is clearly understood [22]. In the vast majority of colorectal cancers,
an adenoma undergoes malignant degeneration. Removing adenomas from the
colon dramatically reduces the risk of colon cancer [23]. If benign adenomas are
removed prior to the development of malignancy, colon cancer is essentially pre-
ventable [24]. The problem is finding benign adenomas. Diagnostic imaging with
air contrast barium enemas or conventional colonoscopy exams has been the primary means by which a clinician searches for adenomas. However, there is a whole
host of issues involving patient compliance and the acceptance of air contrast
barium enema or colonoscopy. Virtual colonoscopy techniques have been introduced as potential methods for colorectal screening and preoperative staging and
combine volumetric imaging based on CT [25, 26, 27] or MR [28, 29] data sets with
sophisticated image processing (Fig. 4). Unfortunately, virtual colonoscopy has
not gained widespread applicability among the medical community.

In only a few minutes, a virtual technique using MSCT can perform a study
that looks inside the colon for adenomatous polyps. This technique is particularly attractive due to the increased potential for patient compliance. A screening
technique for cancer would ideally be cost effective in certain age groups simply
because it is inexpensive, would be interpreted rapidly, and would cost effectively
lower mortality from the cancer.

Screening for colorectal cancer with virtual colonoscopy is well tolerated by
patients, although it does involve a cleansing preparation for the colon. The procedure is safe, and the 3D images are quite compelling and allow for a number of
unique abilities, such as separating out polyps from nodular folds by virtually
splitting the colon open. This ability will hopefully improve the accuracy of diagnoses for adenomatous polyps, making 3D techniques comparable in accuracy
to air contrast barium enema studies. There are critical scanning parameters for
acquiring data for 3D imaging. The data sets for virtual colonoscopy are acquired
using 4 x 1-mm slice collimation, slice thickness 1.25 mm, data reconstruction
interval 1 mm and a pitch of 6.

Different recent studies compared the performance of virtual and conventional colonoscopy for the detection of colorectal polyps [27]. Most groups conclude
that in a population of patients at high risk for colorectal neoplasia, virtual and
conventional colonoscopy had similar efficacy for the detection of polyps that
were 6 mm or more in diameter [26]. Optimal conditions (high-resolution CT
data sets and superior bowel cleansing) allowed researchers to detect relatively
small polyps. These polyps, those around 1 cm in size, are those that physicians

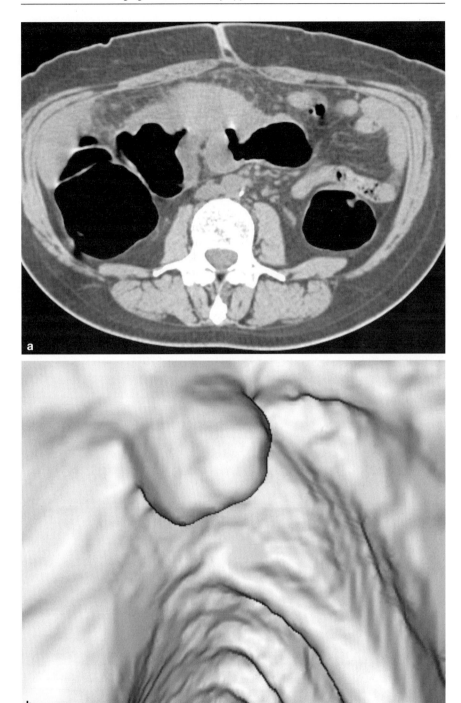

Fig. 4a, b

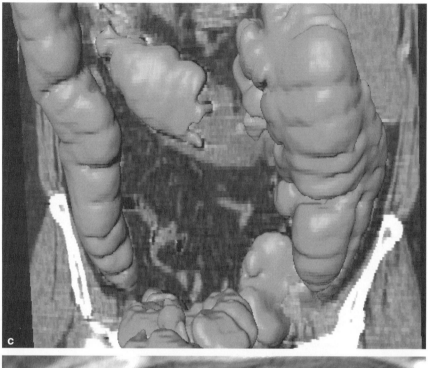

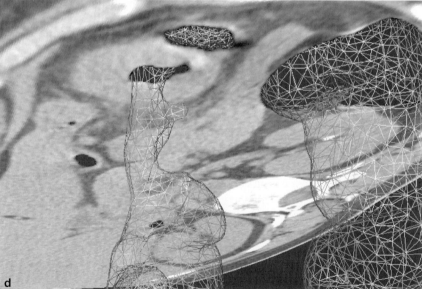

Fig. 4a–d. Nodular folds can mimic polyps even in a two-dimensional mode (2D; **a**), and so the 3D display and virtual endoscopy display (**b**) can help in distinguishing between the two. **c** Two carcinomas in the transverse colon. With this technology, physicians are able to examine areas that colonoscopists cannot. Colonoscopists cannot move their scope through an obstructing lesion (**d**), but this technology can easily see through even a pinhole opening with computed tomography

want to catch before malignant degeneration. Although gastroenterologists would like to find even smaller polyps, the incidence of cancer in a 1-cm polyp is only about two percent.

The problem with earlier 3D images was the time it took to create them. During the time of the first studies, it took almost 2 h to create the endoscopic movies. However, researchers have made significant strides in automating this process in the last 2–3 years. One of the first steps forward in the field of colon cancer research was the creation of an automated path through the colon that recognized the absolute, mathematical epicenter of an air-distended colon. The clinician has only to click on the colon and click on the cecum, and it connects the dots of the pneumocolon view.

In order for this technology to prove cost effective, the time that it takes to interpret these studies must be reasonable. Looking at 300 MSCT sections, even in an endoscopic mode, takes at least 20 min for viewing movies in forward and reverse. An automated solution for initially screening the colon is essential. Programmers and experts in artificial intelligence have been working to develop software that can screen the colon for polyps [30, 31]. It is probably not worth the time it takes to scan through 5 feet of colon in 40 min in order to find one polyp. However, if a smart software program can indicate which areas of the colon are potentially abnormal, then clinicians can direct their efforts to those areas in order to determine whether there truly is a problem.

When a camera is being led along a light source, 360° of the colonic surface cannot be seen due to the limit of the angles and the inevitable blind spots. In order to get around this problem, two things are being done. The patients are being scanned in both supine and prone positions in order to circumvent problems with fluid and with distension of the different segments. In addition, rotating the camera around 360° covers the entire colonic mucosa. Endoscopists cannot see this full a picture, and this technology has found polyps that colonoscopists have missed. Although colonoscopy is a skilled procedure, the view is limited to what can be seen when the scope is retracted; inevitably, there are blind spots. Inadequate distention, fluid, and fecal debris limit the advantages of this virtual technology. However, these limitations also can be partially overcome by looking at supine and prone views and by having the camera look at 100 percent of the colonic mucosa 100 percent of the time. Radiologists using this technology must also look carefully to see whether there is any air within a filling defect of the colon. Even on the endoscopic views, fecal residue can look relatively rounded, and so endoscopic views alone will not suffice; radiologists must refer back to the axial source images.

Virtual Bronchoscopy

Virtual bronchoscopy is emerging as a useful approach for assessment of 3D MSCT pulmonary images. A protocol for virtual bronchoscopic assessment of a MSCT pulmonary image would have two main stages:

1. preprocessing of image data, which involves extracting objects of interest, defining paths through major airways, and preparing the extracted objects for 3D rendering and

2. interactive image assessment, which involves use of graphics-based software
   tools, such as surface-rendered views, projection images, virtual endoscopic
   views, oblique section images, measurement data, and cross-sectional views.

Although a virtual bronchoscope offers a unique opportunity for exploration and
quantitation, it cannot replace a real bronchoscope. Limitations of current VE
systems include high cost, lack of visual aids beyond simulated endoscopic views,
difficulty in performing interactive anatomic exploration, and need for substantial off-line display computation. Future needs include development of fully integrated user-friendly virtual bronchoscopes, development of optimal CT protocols for generating artifact-free data sets, and improvements in automated
preprocessing of 3D CT images. VE reproduces real endoscopic images but cannot provide information on the aspect of the mucosa or biopsy specimens. It
offers possible applications for preparing, guiding, and controlling interventional
fibroscopy procedures.

However, virtual bronchoscopy based on MSCT data permits an investigation
of peripheral bronchi far beyond those that can be examined using a physical
bronchoscope. Indications for virtual bronchoscopy include evaluation of bron-

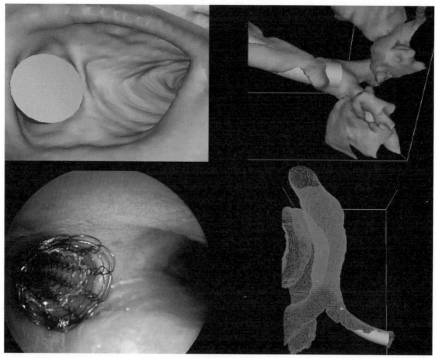

Fig. 5. Virtual bronchoscopy in a patient with stenosis to the bronchi due to masses by Wegener Granulomatosis. A virtual stent is placed in the left main stem bronchus. The three-dimensional simulation during inspiration and during expiration allows for interactive adjustments in course, length,
and in proximal and distal diameters of the virtual device, which can be used as a template for defining the optimal stent configuration

chial anastomosis following lung transplantation, evaluation of abnormalities of the central airways after intubation, tracheotomy, or irradiation of the neck, bronchial stenosis in Wegener granulomatosis, and airway reconstruction after tumor resection [32]. Functional imaging of the tracheobronchial tree is also possible by acquiring a scan in inspiration and in expiration.

Furthermore, the MSCT data can be used to generate an interactive 3D virtual bronchoscopic approach for preoperative endotracheal stent planning [33]. Acquired data are transferred to an independent computer workstation. Once the threshold has been determined, perspective endoluminal renderings of the bronchial tree containing the pathology is performed with a sophisticated software package based on a combination of volume and surface rendering developed and implemented in our 3D lab [33, 34]. The same data can be used to obtain minimum-intensity projections. These are helpful for assessment of location, length, and severity of the airway stenosis. The software allows real-time interpretation of different MPRs simultaneously with interactive VE of the bronchial structures. The system automatically calculates the median centerline of the bronchial lumina. A virtual stent is placed along this generated path (Fig. 5). Subsequently, the software enables interactive adjustments in course, length, and proximal and distal diameters of the virtual device. Once optimized, the virtual device is extracted from the 3D data set as a template for defining the optimal stent configuration.

Surgical Planning and Surgical Simulation

Early attempts to use the wealth of 3D image data to really simulate a surgical plan were limited to cases with symmetric osteotomies, thus limiting the surgical simulation to a 2D cut-move-and-paste task in the lateral aspect to reposition the osseous parts. Complex 3D simulations were difficult to perform with the help of dedicated software only and were first carried out using physical models. Early applications created the ideal end result without simulating the surgery itself. First, surgical simulation was based on wire frames constructed by connecting landmarks that had been extracted from anterior–posterior and lateral cephalograms. Later on, the more complex task of 3D simulation on a display screen was addressed by defining different types of cutting operations that could work in 3D while the user was only watching the 2D display of the 3D image. A first possibility was to draw a cutting line onto the CT-based 3D image or onto simplified derived 3D representations called polygon solid models [35]. Today, most surgical planning applications are based on complex polygonal surface models, where generalized marching cube modules are used for extracting isosurfaces from segmentation results. Orthopedic visualization can take advantage of many of the inherent features for manipulation and measurement in 3D volume imaging for the investigation of skeletal structures in the body. Creation of orthogonal and oblique multi-planar reformatted images permits the orthopedic surgeon to visualize the structure in full context, rather than only in the plane of acquisition, and provides the ability to create images necessary for direct quantitative analysis. 3D rendering techniques are easily applied to the visualization of bone from

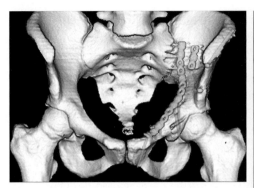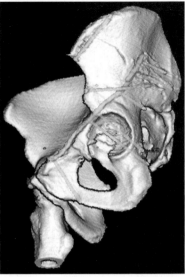

Fig. 6. Complex intra-acetabular fracture. Rendered images from multislice computed tomography data of the hip of a trauma patient after osteosynthesis with cortical screws and reconstruction plates. The intra-acetabular fracture and the related osteosynthesis material cannot be visualized from the initial anterior–posterior rendering. However, by segmenting the head of the femur and translating it away from the hip, the hip can be rotated independently to visualize the acetabular situation clearly. Such high quality three-dimensional reconstructions provide the base for future computer- and robotics-based procedures which will gain increased importance with reduced patient morbidity and improved reconstruction of the joint surface

MSCT data sets, as shown in Figure 6. From CT data, the bone can be segmented using simple thresholding and directly rendered, as shown in this rendering of the pelvis and partial femurs. These renderings are from a patient with an intra-acetabular fracture. The complex fracture cannot be visualized directly from the initial anterior–posterior rendering, and may not be well appreciated in conventional plain films or by reviewing a standard set of transaxial CT sections through this region. Using multiple object segmentation and rendering techniques, the head of the femur can be defined as a separate object and manipulated independently from the pelvis [36]. By subtracting the femur away from the hip, a direct view into the acetabulum can be obtained, providing a view of the fracture to the surgeon otherwise impossible to obtain. In orthopedic applications, it is frequently necessary to understand the soft tissue structures surrounding the skeletal structure of interest. New generations of software packages allow rendering of these soft tissues on top of the underlying skeletal structures, with cutaway sections allowing correlated visualization of the bone and soft tissue.

Another use of surgical planning is the preoperative endoluminal aortic stent planning on a virtual angioscopic rendering system based on MSCTA. The purpose of a recent study was to evaluate an interactive 3D virtual angioscopic approach based on MSCTA data sets of the aorta for preoperative endoluminal aortic stent planning [34]. CTA was performed with the recent generation of MSCT (SOMATOM Volume Zoom, Siemens) with a 4 x 2.5 mm collimation and a pitch of 6. The MSCT data sets of 25 patients with abdominal aortic aneurysms were analyzed with the prototype MedIS application (combination of volume and surface rendering). The software allows for interactive adjustments in

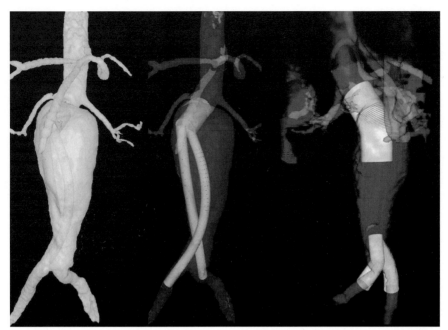

Fig. 7. Advanced software packages based on a combination of volume and surface rendering allow interactive virtual aortoscopy. These systems calculate the optimal centerline of vessel flow lumina. A virtual stent is placed along this generated path. Subsequently, the software allows for adjustments in course, length, and in proximal and distal diameters of the virtual device.
Simulation of the stent within the aorta allows accurate measurements, assuring successful stent placement

course, length and proximal and distal diameters of the virtual device (Fig. 7). The virtual devices are used as templates for defining the optimal stent configurations. The abdominal CT acquisition for a scan volume of 50 cm was performed in 17.8 s and intravenous contrast application was reduced. Simulation of the stent within the aorta provided accurate measurements, assuring successful stent placement in all patients. In contrast to current techniques based on indirect measurements of aortic morphology, this new approach provides direct data of the stent itself. The new MSCT technique provided accurate data for non-invasive preoperative aortoiliac measurements, and the feasibility and advantages of a 3D Virtual Angioscopic Guidance System for optimal planning of intraluminal stent therapy based on MSCTA was demonstrated.

Until now, we have only discussed surgical simulation of rigid bone tissue and standard implants. Simulation of soft tissues is much more complicated but has been attempted on the basis of CT data or the combination of CT and skin digitization. The quality of soft tissue simulation has been recently improved by using MSCT data sets in a variety of applications for surgical planning and surgical simulation. Its major advantages over conventional CT, with higher temporal and spatial resolution, has a very high impact to come close for a perfect surgical simulation. Unlike single-slice CT, in which image acquisition is limited by the scan range and respiration artifacts, MSCT has sufficient speed to obtain thin-section images of the entire body region during peak vascular enhancement. The operator can select parameters, such as collimation and tube current. Thin collimation in combination with perfect timed contrast enhancement produces optimal raw data for soft tissue reconstruction and is therefore likely to become the standard for surgical planning and surgical simulation. In addition, MSCT may prove to be a cost-effective preoperative strategy when compared with the current MR imaging (MRI) applications.

All surgical simulation techniques discussed above are more or less off-line procedures that take considerable time and, if the outcome is not correct, the process has to be repeated. Therefore, the trend is now to devise real-time interactive surgical simulation techniques that can be used both for surgical simulation and for training surgeons, just like the flight simulators used for training professional pilots. Since this process is a virtual surgery, it is related to the computer graphics techniques associated with virtual reality. Virtual reality simulation tries, by the use of head-mounted displays and tracking of hand and instrument motion using a data glove or other interactive devices, to create a simulation that is as realistic as possible. In some cases, there is also sound feedback, and the very important form of feedback for surgeons is tactile or haptic feedback. The most difficult part, again, is the soft-tissue simulation (deformation, cutting characteristics of different organs, and bleeding after cutting) [37]. Different prototype systems for laparoscopic surgical simulation are addressing this issue and will be followed by other systems in the market. Improvement of these systems is expected when they are based on detailed data sets such as that of the visible human project. However, individualized surgery will have to be based on patient-specific data sets from medical imaging modalities, which is today possible with high resolution MSCT data sets. In case these modalities still provide too much data for real-time interaction, techniques are available to drastically reduce the amount of data without significantly violating the morphologic accuracy. The Virtual Reality technology is only emerging and is expected to support, in addition to surgical simulation, many other fields in medicine, such as interactive anatomy education and telepresence surgery. These applications are expected to become essential building blocks of the digital tools used by the physician of this century.

The National Aeronautics and Space Administration (NASA) researchers have developed an immersive virtual environment for the simulation of animal and patient surgeries [38]. NASA is interested in surgical simulations because animal dissection for the scientific examination of organ subsystems as well-performing surgical procedures under the complex environment of microgravity is a challenging task, which is complicated by limited realism afforded by conventional terrestrial training. Their simulation uses the latest techniques for interactive performance, can be run on multiple platforms, and distributed to multiple users. This system allows the user to train for patient surgeries and scientific animal dissections with variations in anatomy and gravitational conditions. Using high-resolution MSCT data sets (Fig. 8a), a real-time, distributed virtual rat simulation system with soft-tissue deformation, force feedback, and variable gravity was demonstrated. This environment allows the surgeon to practice their surgery on

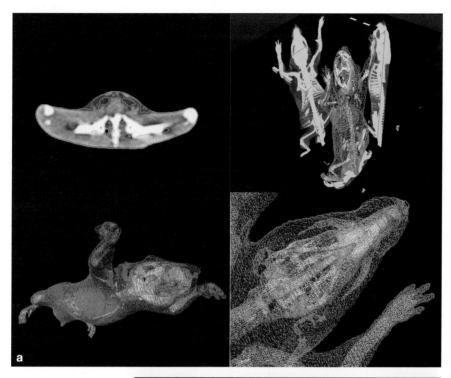

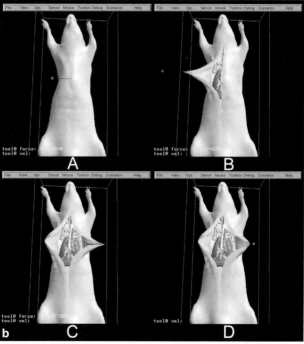

Fig. 8a, b

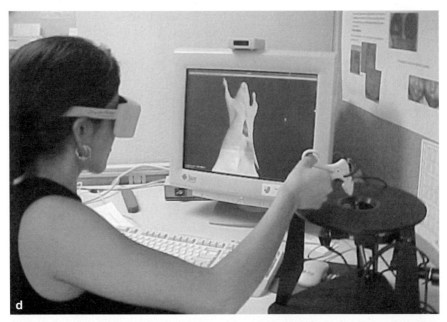

Fig. 8a–c. Using the original multislice computed tomography data set of a small, fully anesthetized rat (0.5-mm collimation, 512 x 512matrix), a high resolution polygonal surface model (**a**) was generated with the resulting mesh of the skin, important internal organs, and bones, consisting of over one million triangles. The mesh was reduced to 100,000 triangles using a mesh simplification module, which is more reasonable for interactive simulations. **b, c** An interactive session with the rat dissection simulator

a computer model of their actual patient and to feel forces as if they were doing the real procedure (Fig. 8a–b). This type of system will be crucial to maintain surgical skills and plan surgeries during long-duration space missions. Many applications in medical education, surgical training, surgical planning, and intra-operative assistance will profit from such systems in the near future.

Conclusions

This article describes, in particular, the methodology of VR and surface rende-ring with some examples. Very often it is asked whether VR or SSD is the more suitable method for the handling of MSCT data sets.

Although many different reconstruction techniques for the handling of volu-metric data sets exists in the field of 3D imaging in combination with MSCT only, VR is mentioned and discussed extensively. VR is, at the moment, surely the most suitable method for handling and visualizing the enormous amount of MSCT data and permits a fast and exact diagnostic assistance for the radiologist in daily routine. Likewise, this method is ideal for presentations.

Some authors focus, however, too strongly on VR only, and it is absolutely incorrect to conclude that surface rendering is obsolete. Most other methods of

3D visualization also profit enormously from the isotropic volume data of MSCT. For example, most research groups in the field of surgical planning, surgical simulation, tissue modeling, and automated lesion detection work mainly with surface rendering methods, respectively polygon-based techniques.

For certain applications, MPR is sufficient. In addition to the best data acquisition technique and the professional image interpretation, the proper selection of the 3D reconstruction method, depending upon clinical question, is also one of the main functions of the radiologist.

Careful attention to technical details in all phases of MSCT, including data acquisition, image processing, and image display, is essential in order to consistently produce optimal 3D studies. A basic understanding of each of these steps helps the radiologist to tailor the examination to specific clinical problems and avoid potential pitfalls. With optimal technique, one 3D reconstruction can provide very accurate images, which obviate the need for multiple conventional 2D images in many circumstances. Continuing advances in scanner and image processing technology promise to further enhance both the accuracy and the practicality of 3D imaging and virtual reality applications.

MSCT, the ability to capture four slices of data with one gantry rotation, increases speed and anatomic coverage. However, just as with the transition from dynamic to helical CT, the software must accompany it. The full impact of the multislice scanner will not be felt until real-time 3D is a reality. The real-time assessment of volumes of data will overcome the limitations of scanning at a thinner collimation. When the virtual reality revolution happens for CT and MR, anatomy will need to be relearned. Clinicians will need to think in terms of volumes and regions of interest rather than 2D axial images, and that is a very exciting prospect, indeed.

References

1. Berland LL, Smith JK (1998) Multidetector-array CT: once again, technology creates new opportunities (editorial; comment). Radiology 209:327–329
2. Klingenbeck-Regn K, et al. (1999) Subsecond multi-slice computed tomography: basics and applications. Eur J Radiol 31:110–124
3. Hu H, et al. (2000) Four multidetector-row helical CT: image quality and volume coverage speed. Radiology 215:55–62
4. Disler DG, Marr DS, Rosenthal DI (1994) Accuracy of volume measurements of computed tomography and magnetic resonance imaging phantoms by three-dimensional reconstruction and preliminary clinical application. Invest Radiol 29:739–745
5. Pfeifer T, et al. (1992) The value of tumor volumetry as opposed to bidimensional determination of tumor size during follow-up of hepatic metastases from colorectal carcinoma. Rofo Fortschr Geb Rontgenstr Neuen Bildgeb Verfahr 157:548–551
6. Horton KM, Fishman EK (2000) 3D CT angiography of the celiac and superior mesenteric arteries with multidetector CT data sets: preliminary observations. Abdom Imaging 25:523–525
7. Glenn WV Jr, et al. (1975) 1975 Memorial award paper. Image generation and display techniques for CT scan data. Thin transverse and reconstructed coronal and sagittal planes. Invest Radiol 10:403–416
8. Lorenson WE, Cline HE (1987) Marching cubes: a high resolution 3D surface construction algorithm. Computer graphics. Proc SIGGRAPH'87 21:163–169
9. Guy RL, et al. (1992) The role of 3D CT in the assessment of acetabular fractures. Br J Radiol 65:384–389
10. Martinez CR, et al. (1992) Evaluation of acetabular fractures with two- and three-dimensional CT. Radiographics 12:227–242

11. Hufner T, et al. (1999) The value of CT in classification and decision making in acetabulum fractures. A systematic analysis. Unfallchirurg 102:124–131
12. Marsh JL, et al. (1986) Applications of computer graphics in craniofacial surgery. Clin Plast Surg 13:441–448
13. Fukuta K, et al. (1990) Three-dimensional imaging in craniofacial surgery: a review of the role of mirror image production. Eur J Plastic Surg 13:209–217
14. Zeman RK, et al. (1995) Diagnosis of aortic dissection: value of helical CT with multiplanar reformation and three-dimensional rendering. AJR Am J Roentgenol 164:1375–1380
15. Calhoun PS, et al. (1999) Three-dimensional volume rendering of spiral CT data: theory and method. Radiographics 19:745–764
16. Pretorius ES, Fishman EK (1999) Volume-rendered three-dimensional spiral CT: musculoskeletal applications. Radiographics 19:1143–1160
17. Vining DJ (1996) Virtual endoscopy: is it reality? Comment on: Radiology 1996 200:49–54. Radiology 200:30–31
18. Robb RA (2000) Virtual endoscopy: development and evaluation using the visible human datasets. Comput Med Imaging Graph 24:133–151
19. Rubin GD, et al. (1996) Perspective volume rendering of CT and MR images: applications for endoscopic imaging. Radiology 199:321–330
20. Schreyer AG, et al. (2000) Virtual CT cystoscopy: color mapping of bladder wall thickness (in process citation). Invest Radiol 35:331–334
21. NCI (1999) Surveillance, epidemiology, and end results (SEER). http://www.seer.ims.nci.nih.gov
22. Vogelstein B, et al. (1988) Genetic alterations during colorectal-tumor development. N Engl J Med 319:525–532
23. Toribara NW Sleisenger MH (1995) Screening for colorectal cancer (see comments). N Engl J Med 332:861–867
24. Winawer SJ, et al. (1996) Prevention of colorectal carcinoma. Current WHO guidelines for early detection of colorectal carcinoma. World Health Organization Collaborating Center for the Prevention of Colorectal Cancer. Leber Magen Darm 26:139–140
25. Vining DJ (1997) Virtual colonoscopy 7:285–291
26. Fenlon HM, et al. (1999) A comparison of virtual and conventional colonoscopy for the detection of colorectal polyps (see comments; published erratum appears in N Engl J Med 2000 342:524). N Engl J Med 341:1496–1503
27. Fletcher JG, Luboldt W (2000) CT colonography and MR colonography: current status, research directions and comparison. Eur Radiol 10:786–801
28. Luboldt W, et al. (1997) Preliminary assessment of three-dimensional magnetic resonance imaging for various colonic disorders 349:1288–1291
29. Luboldt W, et al. (2000) Colonic masses: detection with MR colonography. Radiology 216:383–388
30. Karadi C, et al. (1999) Display modes for CT colonography. Part I. Synthesis and insertion of polyps into patient CT data. Radiology 212:195–201
31. Beaulieu CF, et al. (1999) Display modes for CT colonography. Part II. Blinded comparison of axial CT and virtual endoscopic and panoramic endoscopic volume-rendered studies. Radiology 212:203–212
32. Quint LE, et al. (1995) Stenosis of the central airways: evaluation by using helical CT with multiplanar reconstructions. Radiology 194:871–877
33. Wildermuth S, et al. (2000) Interactive planning system for endobronchial stent placement based on virtual bronchoscopic rendering of multislice CT datasets. (in press)
34. Wildermuth S, et al. (2000) Preoperative endoluminal aortic stent planning on a virtual angioscopic rendering system based on multidetector CT angiography. In ECR. Eur J Radiol 10[suppl]:245
35. Alberti C (1980) Three-dimensional CT and structure models (letter). Br J Radiol 53:261–262
36. Robb RA, Hanson DP, Camp JJ (1996) Computer-aided surgery planning and rehearsal at Mayo Clinic. Computer 29:39–47
37. Satava RM (1995) Medical applications of virtual reality. J Med Syst 19:275–280
38. Bruyns C, Montgomery K, Wildermuth S (2000) Advanced astronaut training/simulation system for rat dissection and surgical simulation. In SMARTSYSTEMS 2000; the International Conference for Smart Systems and Robotics in Space and Medicine. Johnson Space Center, Houston, USA: NASA

II Multislice Computed Tomography in Neuroradiology

Intracranial and Cervical Three-Dimensional Computed Tomography Angiography Using a Multislice Computed Tomography System: Initial Clinical Experience

Yukunori Korogi, Kazuhiro Yoshizumi, Yoshiharu Nakayama, Masataka Kadota, Mutsumasa Takahashi

Abstract. After the introduction of a new multislice computed tomography (MSCT) scanner, it has become possible to produce high-speed CT angiography (CTA) of high quality for the intracranial and cervical vessels. In our initial experience, 66 consecutive patients with known or suspected carotid and/or intracranial arterial lesions underwent CTA using a MSCT scanner. Three scanning techniques were adopted for

1. high-speed CTA covering both cervical and intracranial vessels;
2. high-quality intracranial imaging and high-speed cervical imaging with double injection of contrast materials; and
3. high-quality CTA for intracranial vessels.

A total of 90–105 ml of contrast material (300 mgI, non-ionic) was injected at a rate of 3 ml/s using a power injector. With a MSCT scanner, three-dimensional (3D) CTA images of excellent quality were obtained in all cases without overlapping of cavernous sinuses and intracranial veins because of shorter acquisition time. Approximately 25 cm of scanning extent, enough to cover from the carotid bifurcation to distal cerebral arteries, could be obtained in 16 s with good image quality. In the visualization of small branches, high-speed CTA of high quality was equivalent to intra-arterial digital subtraction angiography (IADSA) and superior to magnetic resonance angiography. The MSCT scanner can provide 3D CTA of excellent quality with significantly shorter acquisition time in the intracranial and cervical regions.

Introduction

There are several applications of MSCT in the field of neuroradiology, including routine CT examination of the head, high-resolution multi-planar reconstruction, or three-dimensional (3D) images, high-speed intracranial and cervical 3D CT angiography (CTA), and high-resolution temporal bone imaging.

After introduction of a new MSCT scanner, it has become possible to produce high-speed CTA of high quality [1, 2]. Although there have been many reports of CTA with MSCT for the aorta and peripheral vessels, its application to the intracranial and cervical vessels has been limited [3]. Therefore, the purpose of this study is to report our initial experience of CTA using a MSCT scanner.

Materials and Methods

Patient Selection

In our initial experience, 66 consecutive patients with known or suspected carotid and/or intracranial arterial lesions underwent CTA using a MSCT scanner. Sixty-six cases [34 males and 32 females; 12–83 years old (mean age 59 years old)] were examined. Twenty-seven patients had cerebral aneurysms, eighteen had arterial occlusive lesions, four had arteriovenous malformations (AVMs)/dural arteriovenous fistulas (AVFs), nine had tumors of the head and neck or intracranial regions, and ten had miscellaneous lesions.

CT technique

The CT units used were LightSpeed QX/I (GEMS) and SOMATOM Plus 4 Volume Zoom (Siemens). We used several scanning methods. For covering both cervical and intracranial arteries, two techniques were applied. Protocol one (high-speed CTA) was performed with 1.25 mm or 2.5 mm slice thickness and pitch 6, and protocol two was performed with double injections of contrast media with intracranial areas scanned first with 1.25 mm slice thickness and pitch 3, followed by cervical regions scanned with 2.5 mm slice thickness and pitch 6.

For intracranial arteries alone, high-quality CTA with 1.25 mm slice thickness and pitch 3 was used. Workstations used included Advantage Windows 3.1 (GEMS) or 3DVirtuoso R2.5.2 (Siemens). Images (3D CTA) were generated from a CT data set using a volume-rendering (VR) algorithm and compared with IADSA and MRA.

Injection of Contrast Media

A total of 90–105 ml of contrast media (300 mgI, non-ionic) was injected at a rate of 3–3.5 ml/s using a power injector. For double-injection method, 60 ml of contrast media was used for each scanning.

Test Injection of Contrast Media for Better Delineation between Arteries and Veins
Images of the arteries on cervical CTA are often degraded due to overlaps of the venous system. To image before the visualization of the venous system, we measure arrival times of contrast media not only at the artery but also at the vein. We inject 20 ml of contrast media for a test injection, CT values of the carotid artery and jugular vein are monitored at the level of the carotid bifurcation, and a time-density curve is drawn. Then, the difference of arrival time between the artery and vein, Δt, is calculated. In clinical scanning for the cervical CTA, the scan parameters are adjusted so as to finish the scanning within Δt in each patient. Overlaps of the veins can be avoided. When only the artery is monitored, however, significant overlap of the jugular vein may be observed.

Results

Comparison of the Two Scanning Techniques

Images of excellent quality were obtained in each case for all scanning techniques without overlapping of the cavernous sinuses and intracranial veins because of shorter acquisition time.

Intracranial and Cervical CTA: Protocol One

Approximately 30 cm of scanning extent, enough to cover from the carotid bifurcation to distal cerebral arteries, could be obtained in 16 s with good image quality (Fig. 1). Opacification of the jugular vein was minimal, while the intracranial venous systems were seen.

Intracranial and Cervical CTA: Protocol Two

In comparison with protocol one, images of the intracranial arteries of better image quality were obtained and the cervical veins were less visualized (Fig. 2). However, a larger amount of contrast media was necessary in this technique.

Intracranial and Cervical 3D CTA

Arterial Occlusive Lesions

Screening of the arterial occlusive lesions is routinely done with Doppler US or MRA. Advantages of 3D CTA with MSCT include a large field of view that is particularly useful for the tandem lesions, short examination time, detection of cal-

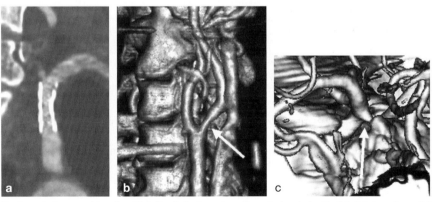

Fig. 1a–c. A 64-year-old male with left subclavian artery stenosis (post stenting), left internal carotid artery stenosis, and right internal carotid-posterior communicating artery aneurysm (computed tomography angiography: 1.25-mm slice thickness, pitch 6, scan length 295 mm, and scan time 31.5 s). **a** Multi-planar reconstruction image of the left subclavian artery shows patent lumen at the stenting site. **b** Volume rendering (VR) image of the left internal carotid artery shows mild narrowing (*arrow*). **c** VR image of the small right internal carotid artery aneurysm (*arrow*). All images could be obtained during one scan. This technique is useful for the patients with multiple vascular lesions like in this patient

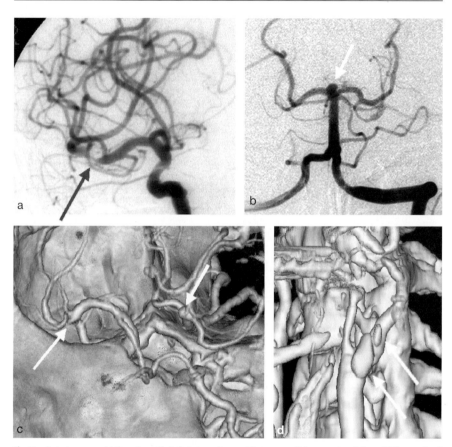

Fig. 2a–d. A 64-year-old female with left internal carotid artery mild stenosis, right middle cerebral artery stenosis, tip of the basilar artery aneurysm (computed tomography angiography: 1.25-mm slice thickness, pitch 3 for intracranial and 2.5-mm slice thickness, pitch 6 for cervical region). **a** Intra-arterial digital subtraction angiography (IADSA) of the right carotid angiogram shows a stenosis of the right middle cerebral artery (*arrow*). **b** IADSA of the vertebral angiogram shows an aneurysm at the tip of the basilar artery (*arrow*). **c** Volume rendering (VR) image clearly demonstrates both stenosis and aneurysm (*arrows*) **d** VR image of the cervical carotid artery shows calcifications

cification, and evaluation of the post-treatment states, such as carotid endarterectomy (CEA) and stenting (Fig. 1 and Fig. 2).

Cerebral Aneurysms

Conventional angiography is still the standard of reference. MRA may be the technique of the first screening, and CTA can be used for the second screening. We have reported the diagnostic accuracy of 3D CTA for the cerebral aneurysms [4] (Fig. 1, Fig. 2 and Fig. 3). Mean sensitivities of CTA in this blinded reader study were 64% (<3 mm), 83% (3–4 mm), 95% (5–12 mm), and 100% (>13 mm) for very small, small, medium, and large aneurysms, respectively. In the diagnosis of the

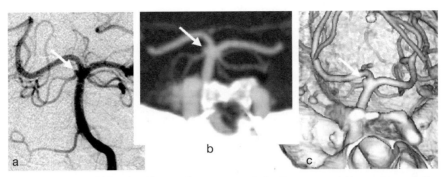

Fig. 3a–c. A 54-year-old female with a small aneurysm at the basilar artery – right superior cerebellar artery bifurcation (computed tomography angiography: 1.25-mm slice thickness, and pitch 3). **a** Intra-arterial digital subtraction angiography shows a very small aneurysm (*arrow*). **b** Maximum intensity projection image from CTA. **c** Volume rendering image. Both CTA images demonstrate the small aneurysm very well (*arrows*)

cerebral aneurysms, the advantages of CTA over MRA include decreased imaging time, less image impairment from the patient motion, compatibility for intubated patients and patients having ferromagnetic intracranial vascular clip, and less likelihood of missing aneurysms with low or turbulent flow.

Brain AVMs

MRA often fails to demonstrate the nidus and draining veins if the contrast media is not used. Also, a multi-slub technique, such as multiple overlapping thin-slab acquisition (MOTSA), is necessary in order to cover the whole AVM components, which results in longer examination time. In contrast, highspeed CTA with MSCT is useful for brain AVM because of larger scanning width (Fig. 4). A 3D VR image can offer better delineation of the complex AVM anatomy. However, hemodynamics in the AVM/AVF cannot be assessed.

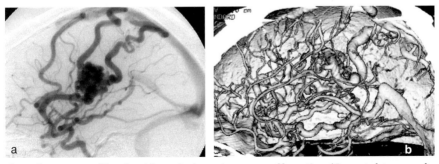

Fig. 4a, b. A 33-year-old male with cerebral arteriovenous malformation. (Computed tomography angiography: 1.25-mm slice thickness, pitch 3, scan length 95 mm, and scan time 25.3 s). **a** Intra-arterial digital subtraction angiography shows brain AVM with dilated draining veins. **b** Volume rendering image of CTA offers better delineation of the complex AVM anatomy with wide view

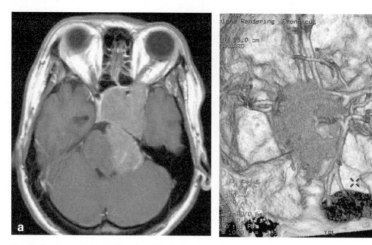

Fig. 5a, b. A 33-year-old female with huge pituitary adenoma. **a** Gadolinium-enhanced T1-weighted image shows large pituitary adenoma that extends into the middle and posterior fossa. **b** Volume rendering image demonstrates the relationship between the tumor and vessels

Brain Tumors

In the well-enhanced mass or skull base tumors, relationships between the tumor and adjacent vessels and tumor and bone may be assessed using CTA with MSCT (Fig. 5).

Conclusion

Advantages of cervical and intracranial CTA with MSCT include high resolution images with a large scan width, shorter imaging time, and lower amount of contrast media. However, a large amount of imaging data should be manipulated and stored. A high quality work station is mandatory and extensive time and labor are needed for postprocessing. Also, use of MSCT may increase radiation exposure because of a large field of view.

Various 3D images obtained from a CTA data set using MSCT are diagnostically useful for preoperative and postoperative evaluation of the vascular diseases and tumors. The MSCT scanner can provide 3D CTA of excellent quality with significantly shorter acquisition time for the intracranial and cervical regions.

References

1. Hu H (1999) Multi-slice helical CT: scan and reconstruction. Med Phys 26:5–18
2. Rubin GD et al. (1999) Computed tomographic angiography: historical perspective and new state-of-the-art using multi detector-row helical computed tomography. JCAT 23:83–90
3. Marks MP (1998) CT angiography of the head and neck. RSNA categorical course in vascular imaging. Radiol Soc North Am, pp 105–109
4. Korogi Y, Takahashi M, Katada K, et al. (1999) Intracranial aneurysms: detection with three-dimensional CT angiography with volume rendering-comparison with conventional angiographic and surgical findings. Radiology 211:497–506

Multislice Spiral Computed Tomography of the Skull Base

Ulrich Baum, Bernd Tomandl, Michael Lell, Matthias Duetsch,
Knut Eberhardt, Holger Greess, Werner Bautz

Introduction

Due to the high spatial resolution and the excellent capability of imaging of osseous structures, computed tomography (CT) is of great importance for the diagnosis of pathologic changes of the skull base. CT is the method of choice for the diagnostic evaluation of fractures and middle ear diseases, such as middle ear hearing loss and anomalies [3]. Examination in transverse and coronal plane is necessary for the detection of discrete lesions.

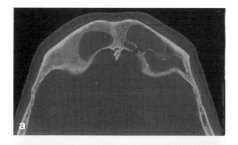

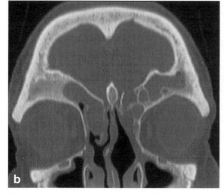

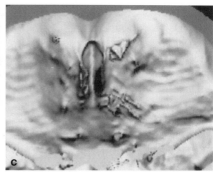

Fig. 1a–c. Mucocele. An 80-year-old male patient with pyoceles of both frontal sinuses (2 years ago) and actual cerebrospinal fluid (CSF) rhinorhea. Multislice spiral computed tomography was performed with a slice collimation of 4 x 1 mm. Interruption of the posterior wall of the left frontal sinus. Hypersclerosis of the bone above the right orbital cavity caused by chronic osteomyelitis after pyocele of the frontal sinuses. Axial plane (**a**), coronal multi-planar reformation (MPR; **b**), surface-shaded display (SSD; **c**)

CT allows the exact depiction of fracture lines in the petrous bone or the anterior cranial fossa. Common complications, such as fracture of the facial canal or the semicircular canals can be visualized using CT [6]. In contrast, pathologies of the inner ear, the internal auditory canal, and the cerebello-pontine angle are preferably examined using magnetic resonance imaging (MRI) [3]. For the evaluation of the petrous apex, CT and MRI are complementary techniques [3]. Further indication for CT of the petrous bone is the preoperative planning and postoperative control of cochlea implants (Fig. 1) [5, 9].

The anterior cranial fossa is the osseous border between the nasopharyngeal space and the frontal lobes. Primary osseous lesions, e.g., congenital variations and anomalies (e.g., craniostenosis), primary and secondary osseous tumors (e.g., osteoma and metastases), inflammatory changes (e.g., mucoceles and pyoceles), and fractures of the frontobasis are often found in this region. The role of diagnostic imaging is to detect or exclude infiltration of the skull base by intracranial (e.g., meningiomas) or nasopharyngeal tumors. The assessment of intratumoral calcifications helps to further characterize the lesions (e.g., craniopharyngioma).

Examination Technique with Single-Slice Spiral CT

Usually, the examination is performed in the transverse plane, in 15–20° angle to the orbitomeatal level. To delineate the skull base, the orbital cavity, the nasopharynx, and the paranasal sinuses, the examination is performed in the coronal plane with hyperextension of the cervical spine. The plane should be in a 70° angle to the orbitomeatal level, perpendicular to the clivus. Some indications [e.g., cholesteatoma, cerebrospinal fluid (CSF) rhinorhea, and abnormalities of the auditory ossicles] require the examination both in the transverse and the coronal plane.

Limitations of Single-Slice Spiral CT

Thin slices are necessary for imaging of osseous structures. Evaluation of the petrous bone, e.g., the auditory ossicles and the inner ear, require high-resolution images with a slice width of 1.0 mm or less. Thicker slices with a higher signal to noise ratio are better suited for soft tissue imaging. For the assessment of soft tissue lesions 2–3 mm thick slices are usually considered a good choice, because thinner slices are too noisy. Single-slice spiral CT therefore requires a compromise between dose, slice collimation, spatial resolution, and the signal to noise ratio for soft tissue images. The quality of secondary reconstructions is limited. Discrete lesions of the roof of the tympanic cavity, the auditory ossicles, or the cribriform plate can hardly be distinguished from artifacts. Coronal scans of the nasal cavity and the paranasal sinuses suffer from beam-hardening artifacts from dental implants and motion artifacts due to the uncomfortable patient positioning with hyperextension of the cervical spine (Fig. 2).

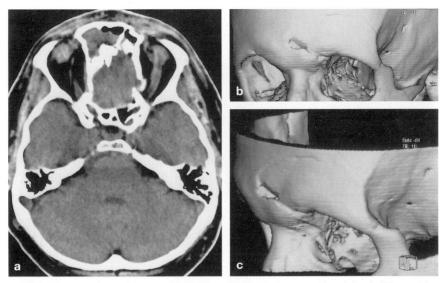

Fig. 2a–c. Fracture of the skull base. Multislice spiral computed tomography of the skull base with a slice collimation of 4 x 1 mm. Soft tissue images of the posterior cranial fossa with a slice width of 4 mm (**a**). Surface-shaded display images (**b, c**) from images with a slice width of 1.25 mm and a reconstruction increment of 0.8 mm. Exclusion of intracranial hematoma on the soft tissue images. Fractures of the cribriform plate, the roof of the tympanic cavity, and the anterior and posterior laminas of the frontal sinuses on the left side. Hematosinus of the ethmoidal sinuses

Improvements of the SOMATOM Volume Zoom for Imaging of the Skull Base

The aim of new CT techniques should be to decrease slice collimation and to increase in-plane resolution as a prerequisite for improved image quality and increased spatial resolution of secondary reconstructions. In comparison with conventional single-slice CT scanners, the multislice spiral CT SOMATOM Volume Zoom (Siemens, Erlangen, Germany) provides considerably increased spatial resolution in the scan plane [2% modulation transfer function (MTF) 22 lp/cm] and in the plane perpendicular to it (by applying 0.5 mm slice width). The reduction of the minimal slice collimation from 1.0 mm to 0.5 mm increases the spatial resolution in longitudinal axis and is therefore the prerequisite for optimized two-dimensional (2D) and 3D reconstructions.

Special techniques (e.g., simultaneous use of both quarter detector offset and flying focal spot; decrease of the effective detector aperture by partially covering the detector elements) can be used to increase in-plane resolution [7]. Using these techniques, the spatial resolution for the SOMATOM Volume Zoom can be increased from 14 lp/cm to 22 lp/cm (2% MTF). This special mode is suitable for the assessment of very small or thin osseous structures, e.g., the petrous bone or the skull base. However, the scan field of view is limited to 25 cm. This scan field of view is large enough to examine the head using a special head support at the end of the examination table.

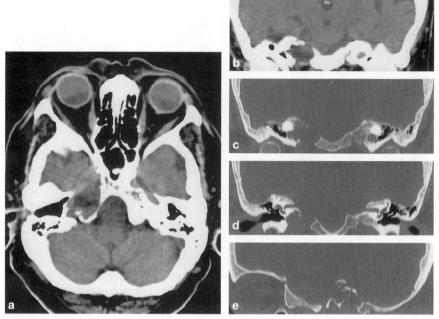

Fig. 3a–e. Histiocytosis X. Multislice spiral computed tomography with a slice collimation of 4 x 10 mm. Osteolytic lesion of the petrous apex on the right side with destruction of the superior and inferior osseous laminas but intact osseus laminas to the inner and the middle ear. Soft tissue images in axial plane (**a**) and coronal plane (**b**). High-resolution multi-planar reformation (MPR) in coronal (**c, d**) and sagittal plane (**e**)

Examination Technique with the SOMATOM Volume Zoom

Depending on the expected pathology (diseases of the bone or the soft tissue) and the origin of the disease (intracranial, skull base, nasopharynx, or orbital cavity), we use different examination protocols (Fig. 3).

Intracranial or Intraorbital Lesion with Suspected Infiltration of the Skull Base

Whereas intracranial lesions with infiltration of the skull base require an examination of the entire neurocranium, the scan volume can be limited to the orbital cavity and the skull base for suspected lesions in the orbital cavity. The examination is performed according to the protocol in Table 1. For the examination of tumors, application of contrast material (c.m.) is mandatory. For secondary reconstructions, the spiral should be reconstructed twice. For assessment in the scan plane and secondary reconstruction, 3-mm and 1.25-mm slices, respectively, are necessary (Table 1).

Table 1. Multislice spiral computed tomography protocol for intracranial tumors with suspected infiltration of the skull base

Scan parameter		
Scan length (mm)	140	
Scan direction	Caudocranial	
Slice collimation (mm)	4x1	
Table feed (mm/rotation)	2.7	
Rotation time (s)	1.0	
Contrast material protocol		
Volume (ml)	100	
Flow rate (ml/s)	1.5	
Start delay (s)	100	
Image reconstruction	Bone	Soft tissue
Slice width (mm)	1.0	3/1.25
Reconstruction increment (mm)	0.5	3/0.5
Slice width (MPR; mm)	1.0	-/3.0
Kernel	High-resolution	Standard

MPR, multi-planar reformation; –, not determined

Petrous Bone/Skull Base

On the SOMATOM Volume Zoom, the examination of the petrous bone and the skull base is performed with the high-resolution protocol in Table 2. For the differentiation between cholesteatoma, chronic otitis media, or malignant tumor, we inject intravenous c.m. Whereas cholesteatoma shows no enhancement after c.m. injection, chronic otitis media and malignant tumors usually enhance after application of c.m.

The image reconstruction of the petrous bone is done with a small field of view (approximately 70–100 mm) for each side. Additionally, coronal images are reconstructed. To reduce noise, the slice width of the multi-planar reformation (MPR) should be 0.5–0.8 mm for the bone and 2–3 mm for the soft tissue images (Table 2).

Table 2. Multislice spiral computed tomography protocol for the skull base and the petrous bone

Scan parameter	
Scan length (mm)	50
Scan direction	Caudocranial
Slice collimation (mm)	2x0.5 (UHR)
Table feed (mm/rotation)	1.0
Rotation time (s)	0.75
Contrast material protocol	
Volume (ml)	120
Flow rate (ml/s)	2.5
Start delay (s)	80
Image reconstruction	
Slice width (mm)	0.5
Reconstr. increment (mm)	0.3
Slice width (MPR; mm)	0.5–0.8
Kernel	UHR

UHR, ultra high-resolution; MPR, multi-planar reformation

Table 3. Multislice spiral computed tomography protocol nasopharyngeal space

Scan parameter		
Scan length (mm)	250	
Scan direction	Craniocaudal	
Slice collimation (mm)	4x1	
Table feed (mm/rotation)	4.0	
Rotation time (s)	0.5	
Contrast material protocol		
Volume (ml)	120	
Flow rate (ml/s)	2.5	
Start delay (s)	80	
Image reconstruction	Soft tissue	Bone
Slice width (mm)	3/1.25	1.0
Reconstruction increment (mm)	3/0.5	0.5
Slice width (MPR; mm)	–/3.0	1.0
Kernel	Standard	High-resolution

MPR, multi-planar reformation

Nasopharyngeal Space

Nasopharyngeal carcinomas are often detected in extensively spread stages with infiltration of the skull base. The examination is performed from the skull base to the aortic arch to delineate bone destruction and to cover all cervical lymph nodes. Intravenous c.m. is mandatory to delineate the tumor from the surrounding soft tissue (Table 3). For exact assessment of the tumor extent and spread, coronal and sagittal reconstructions (bone and soft tissue) are used (Table 3).

Clinical Results and Discussion

Imaging the temporal bone demands high standards. Maximal spatial resolution is necessary to detect discrete pathologic changes. The available spatial resolution of 14 lp/cm (2% MTF) may hinder the detection of discrete changes of the mastoid cells, the middle ear, the inner ear, and early stage tumor infiltration. The described special techniques implemented in the SOMATOM Volume Zoom provides considerably increased spatial resolution in the scan plane. Relative to 1.0-mm slices without ultra high-resolution mode (2% MTF 14 lp/cm), 1.0-mm slices with ultra high-resolution mode (2% MTF 22 lp/cm) significantly improve the delineation of the osseous structures of the petrous bone [1] (Fig. 4 and Fig. 5). The image quality of a MPR out of a 1-mm spiral data set is not always satisfactory. In the past, additional coronal scans were performed to resolve this dilemma.

Compared with 1.0-mm slices, partial volume effects can be further reduced by using slice widths of 0.5 mm. Although the signal to noise ratio decreases, thinner slices result in a better delineation of the auditory ossicles, the cochlea, and the semicircular ducts in the transverse images. In the secondary reconstructions (reconstruction increment 0.3 mm for both the 1.0 mm and the 0.5 mm slices, slice width of the secondary reconstructions 0.7 mm), the overall image quality increased [2]. Usually, critical structures, such as the roof of the tympanic

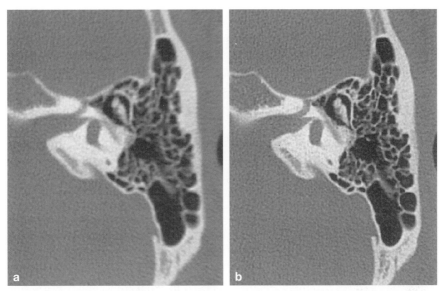

Fig. 4a, b. Comparison of in-plane resolution. Multislice spiral computed tomography of the petrous bone. Comparison of scan modes with different in-plane resolution. Relative to the standard scan reconstructed with a high resolution kernel (**a**), the examination of the petrous bone with the ultra high-resolution scan mode (**b**) allows better delineation of the malleoincudal joint, the canal for the facial nerve, the mastoid, and the internal auditory canal

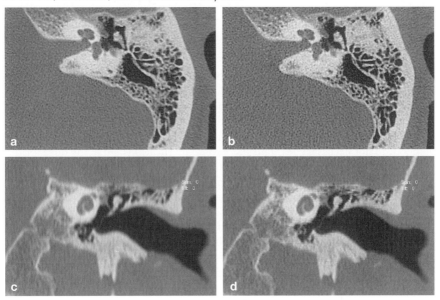

Fig. 5a–d. Comparison of slice width. Multislice spiral computed tomography of the petrous bone with ultra high-resolution scan mode and a slice collimation of 2x0.5 mm. Reconstruction with different slice widths of 1.0 mm (**a, c**) and 0.5 mm (**b, d**). Reconstruction increment 0.3 mm for both. For the multi-planar reformation (MPR), we used a slice width of 0.7 mm. Slightly increased image quality in the axial images with 0.5 mm (Fig. 5a, b), but clearly sharper delineation of the roof of the tympanic cavity, the incus, and the cochlea in the MPR from the data set with a slice width of 0.5 mm (**c, d**)

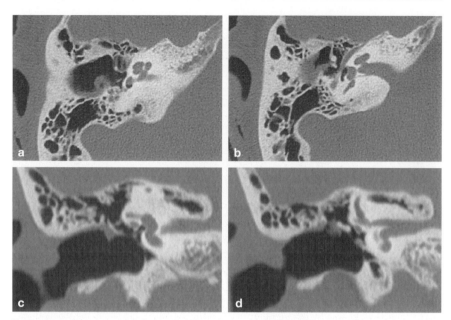

Fig. 6a–d. Cholesteatoma with fixation of the auditory ossicles. Multislice spiral computed tomogra-phy of the petrous bone with ultra high-resolution scan mode and a slice collimation of 2 x 0.5 mm. Small tumor in the epitympanic recess with fixation of the malleolus and the incus. The contact over a long distance is more difficult to see on transverse images (**a, b**) than on the multi-planar reformati-ons (MPRs; **c, d**). Clear delineation of the roof of the tympanic cavity without tumor infiltration

cavity, the incus, or the facial canal, can be assessed without loss of image quality or resolution in any given plane [8]. This helps to define critical relationships of a fracture to the cranial nerves canals, the inner or the middle ear. Curved MPR, for example, allow the presentation of the intraosseous course of the facial nerve in a single image only. In most cases, an additional examination in the coronal plane is therefore not necessary [8]. This has several implications. First, the dose for the lens and the thyroid gland can be reduced. Second, motion artifacts can be mini-mized due to the comfortable supine position of the patient. Third, dental arti-facts do not impair image quality because they are outside the scan volume (Fig. 6 and Fig. 7). The same scan protocol can also be used for examination of osseous structures of the anterior cranial fossa and the craniocervical junction.

For the assessment of tumor extent, the possibility of reconstructing different slice widths from the same data set is a further advantage of multislice spiral CT. While thin slices are used for bone imaging, thicker slices with a better signal to noise ratio can be used for soft tissue imaging. High-resolution multi-planar reconstructions allow the exact assessment of tumor localization, infiltration into the skull base, and lymph node metastases [4]. Discrete changes of the osseous structures within the scan plane, such as the roof of the tympanic cavity or the cribriform plate, can be visualized in any given plane (Fig. 8).

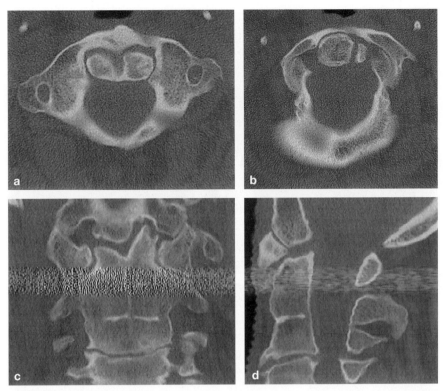

Fig. 7a–d. Anomaly of the craniocervical junction. Multislice spiral computed tomography with the ultra high-resolution scan mode and a slice collimation of 2 x 0.5 mm. Incomplete fusion of the caudal ossification centers of the dens axis. Fusion the cranial ossification center with the clivus. Fusion of the body of the second and the third cervical vertebra. Axial plane (**a, b**), coronal multiplanar reformation (MPR; **c**), and sagittal plane (**d**)

Conclusion

In conclusion, multislice spiral CT SOMATOM Volume Zoom allows the examination of the skull base with substantially improved 3D spatial resolution. Submillimeter high-resolution CT is approaching the goal of isotropic voxels and is thus optimizing imaging quality of the skull base and the temporal bone. Slices with a width of 0.5 mm make additional coronal scans unnecessary and allow the generation of reconstructions not only in the coronal or the transverse plane but also in the sagittal plane or any other desired, e.g., along anatomic structures (e.g., canal of the facial nerve) without loss of image quality.

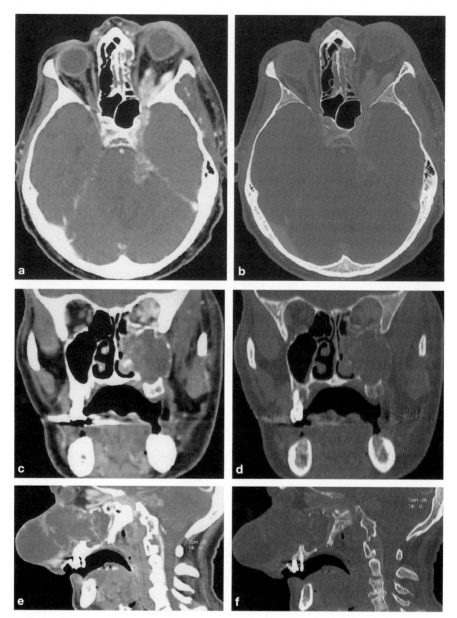

Fig. 8a–e. Malignant melanoma. Multislice spiral computed tomography is performed with a slice collimation of 4 x 1 mm. Large central necrotic tumors in the midface with destruction of the orbital floor and the medial wall of the orbital cavity (**b, c, f**). Hypervascular tumor along the optical nerve (**a, c, e**)

References

1. Baum U, Greess H, Wolf H, Flohr T, Süß C, Lenz M, Kalender WA, Bautz W (1999) Ultrahochauf-lösende Felsenbeindiagnostik mit einem neuen Mehrzeilen-Spiral-CT. Röfo 170[suppl]:4
2. Baum U, Lell M, Noemayr A, Greess H, Wolf H, Tomandl B, Bautz W (2000) Ultrahochauflösende Diagnostik des Felsenbeines mit einem Mehrzeilen-Spiral-CT (MSCT). Röfo 172[suppl]:151
3. Casselman JW (1996) Temporal bone imaging. Neuroimaging Clin North Am 6:265–289
4. Lell M, Baum U, Köster M, Nömayr A, Greess H, Lenz M, Bautz W (1999) Morphologische und funk-tionelle Diagnostik der Kopf-Halsregion mit der Mehrzeilen-Spiral-CT. Radiologe 39:932–938
5. Maher N, Becker H, Laszig R (1995) Quantifizierung relevanter Meßgrößen des Felsenbeins im Computertomogramm vor Cochlear-Implant-Operation. Laryngorhinootologie 74:337–342
6. Marangos N, Berlis A (1995) Hochauflösendes Computertomogramm der Felsenbeine im Kno-chenalgorithmus und 2D-Rekonstruktion zur Beurteilung des Fazialiskanales. HNO 43:732–736
7. Ohnesorge BM, Flohr T, Kopp AF, Baum U, Bae KT (1999) High resolution imaging with multislice spiral CT. Radiology 231[suppl]:318
8. Venema HW, Phao S, Mirek P, Hulsman F, Majoie C, Verbeeten B (1999) Petrosal bone: coronal reconstructions from axial spiral CT data obtained with 0.5 mm collimation can replace direct coronal sequential CT scans. Radiology 213:375–382
9. Wooley AL, Oser AB, Lusk RP, Bahadori RS (1997) Preoperative temporal bone computed tomo-graphy scan and its use in evaluating the pediatric cochlear implant candidate. Laryngoscope 107:1110–1106

III Cardiovascular Multislice Computed Tomography

Cardiac Imaging with Multislice Spiral Computed Tomography

Scan and Reconstruction Principles and Quality Assurance

Willi A. Kalender, Stefan Ulzheimer, Marc Kachelriess

Abstract. Subsecond multislice spiral CT offers high potential for phase-selective and quantitative imaging of the heart and the coronary arteries. We have developed new electrocardiogram (ECG)-based reconstruction algorithms and applied them to data acquired with a Siemens SOMATOM Volume Zoom. Two classes of algorithms were investigated: 180°MCD (multislice cardio delta), a partial scan reconstruction of 180°+δ with δ< fan angle and 180°MCI (multislice cardio interpolation), a piecewise linear interpolation between successive spiral data segments, i.e., successive measured slices and gantry rotations. Effective scan times as low as 56 ms can be achieved with 0.5 s rotation time and $M=4$ simultaneously measured slices for pitch values that allow the coverage of the complete heart during one breath hold. To validate such algorithms, but also to compare arbitrary scanners and scan protocols, we specified and built dedicated quality control phantoms for cardiac CT. The phantom's anthropomorphic body can hold different inserts for calibration purposes (calibration insert) and for the assessment of image quality with moving objects (motion insert). The calibration insert contains calcifications of different sizes and densities of calcium hydroxyapatite (HA). The motion insert consists of a small water tank with different objects attached to water-equivalent rods moving on realistic paths and velocities inside the tank. Calcium objects attached to the rod can be used to compare reproducibility in calcium scoring and to perform resolution tests for moving objects. Three-dimensional (3D) paths and velocities are freely programmable on a PC which also generates the appropriate ECG signal to be used for prospective cardiac triggering or to synchronize retrospective cardiac gating techniques, such as 180°MCD and 180°MCI. Effective scan times of below 100 ms have been verified for the Volume Zoom with 180°MCI in phantom experiments and patient scans. Even for tachycardic situations (>100 bpm) and irregular pulse frequencies, 180°MCI performs very well. The freely programmable motion phantom in combination with the calibration phantom provide excellent tools to compare results for different modalities. The reproducibility for coronary calcium scoring was found to be significantly improved with the SOMATOM Volume Zoom and 180°MCI relative to electron beam CT (EBCT). The tools described appear adequate; a consensus on test procedures and criteria is still necessary.

Introduction

Due to the permanent motion of the heart during data acquisition, standard computed tomography (CT) scanning often results in images with high artifact content and only limited diagnostic use. For typical heart frequencies of 60–120 bpm, the duration of one cardiac cycle is in the range of 0.5 s–1.0 s, i.e., in the range of the rotation times of modern CT scanners. This often results in images representing all cardiac phases superimposed in a mixed form with varying degrees of artifacts. Although some images may look adequate, others do not. There is no consistency; this lack is revealed most clearly in multi-planar reformations (MPR) along the z-axis.

Subsecond scanning with multislice spiral CT offers a high potential for improvements in cardiac imaging. Algorithms have been developed which use only short spiral segments or make use of ECG information in z-interpolation to provide images which present the heart in one motion phase only and therefore with greatly reduced effects due to motion. An example is shown in Figure 1. Early results for these techniques were presented by our group at the fourth SOMATOM Plus User Conference in Rotterdam in 1998 [1]. Cardiac imaging using CT has reached a high standard by now.

Coronary calcium measurements, which are often referred to as "coronary calcium scoring" in the literature, are a particular aim. They have been performed on electron beam CT (EBCT) scanners for many years. Nevertheless, the procedure cannot be considered mature or established. There are no statements on accuracy in clinical work. Accuracy, however, may be considered less important. Reproducibility is more important; it has been specified with approximately 30% for EBCT [2]. Applying the "3σ"rule, this means that a change in patient status can only be diagnosed with certainty if the measured value has changed by at least 80–100%. For a test which is expected to provide high sensitivity, this is

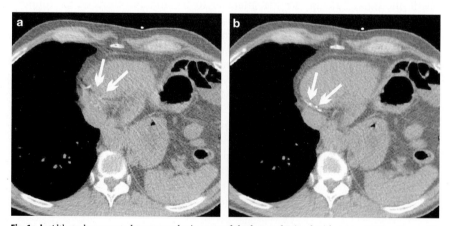

Fig. 1a, b. Although computed tomography images of the heart obtained with 0.5 s rotation time exhibit a low artifact content, many details, such as the calcified coronary artery, are not displayed sharply in a standard reconstruction (**a**). Electrocardiogram-correlated z-interpolation improves this situation significantly (**b**)

completely unacceptable. The reproducibility of the measurement procedure has to be greatly improved and must be assured by appropriate quality control procedures. In addition, the means for a comparison of results obtained with different scanners and scan modes have to be established. Respective proposals will be presented here.

Scanning Techniques and Reconstruction Principles

For cardiac CT applications, it is generally true that the table feed per heart beat should not exceed the total collimation width $M \cdot S$, where the time interval per heart beat is given by the inverse heart frequency $1/f_H$. The parameter M denotes the number of simultaneously acquired slices and S denotes the collimated slice width. The maximum table speed, given by dividing the table increment d by the rotation time t_{rot}, is then given by

$$d' = \frac{d}{t_{rot}} \leq \frac{M \cdot S}{1/f_H}.$$

Consequently, the table feed per rotation and the pitch are restricted as follows:

$$p = \frac{d}{M \cdot S} \leq f_H \cdot t_{rot}.$$

This implies that for spiral CT of the heart, the pitch is limited to relatively small values. For a rotation time of 0.5 s and a heart frequency $f_H=60$ bpm, a maximum pitch of 0.5 results and for $f_H=120$ bpm, a maximum value of 1.0 results.

The ECG is recorded simultaneously with the CT measurement in order to be able to correlate cardiac motion with the measured CT data. The user may define data ranges relative to the ECG which are 'allowed' and can be accessed for reconstruction (Fig. 2a). Such ranges are typically selected relative to the R-waves of the ECG signal; for example, the user can center the allowed ranges at 70% of the R-R intervals.

Two classes of algorithms have been developed, 180°CD (cardio delta) and 180°CI (cardio interpolation) and their respective generalizations 180°MCD (multislice cardio delta) and 180°MCI (multislice cardio interpolation) for single- and multislice spiral CT, respectively [3, 4]. The algorithms 180°CD and 180°MCD use projection data over a range 180+δ ($\delta<$ fan angle) for the reconstruction of a partial scan from the spiral data (Fig. 2b). For cardiac imaging, δ extends to typically 20°; the effective scan time is then approximately 55% of the rotation time t_{rot}. For a physical rotation time of 0.5 s, for example, effective scan times of about 275 ms result; the limit of 250 ms holds true for the center of rotation. This procedure allows a significant reduction of the motion artifacts. The slice sensitivity profile is defined exactly in this case. For higher heart frequencies, i.e., when the motion phases of the heart and the diastolic phase in particular are shorter than the effective scan time, there will be some deterioration of the image quality.

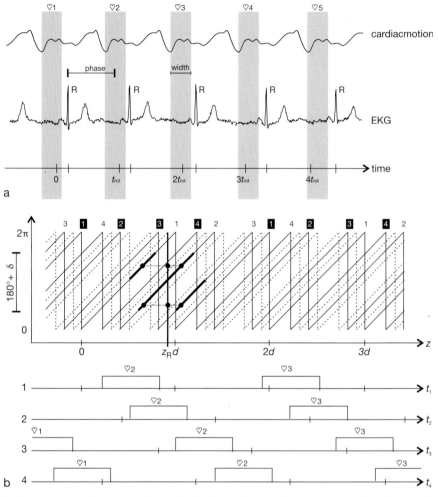

Fig. 2a–c. Electrocardiogram (ECG)-correlated z-interpolation. **a** The ECG is recorded synchronously with the computed tomography measurement. The user selects, relative to the R-waves of the ECG, which data ranges are to be accessed for heart phase-oriented image reconstruction. **b** The algorithm 180°MCD (multislice cardio delta) represents a partial scan reconstruction using a data range of only slightly more than 180°. Effective scan times are approximately 250 ms for a 0.5 s rotation time. **c** The algorithm 180°MCI (multislice cardio interpolation) implies the usual z-interpolation; however, only data from allowed ranges selected in the ECG will be used. The effective scan time is reduced significantly

The algorithms 180°CI and 180°MCI utilize the information from the simultaneously recorded ECG to ensure that only data acquired during the selected heart phase are used for interpolation (Fig. 2c). They also allow a significant reduction of effective scan times, since short intervals of the ECG curve are sufficient in most cases; effective scan times of less than 100 ms can be obtained on a 0.5 s scanner for many heart frequencies as will be demonstrated below [5]. A minor

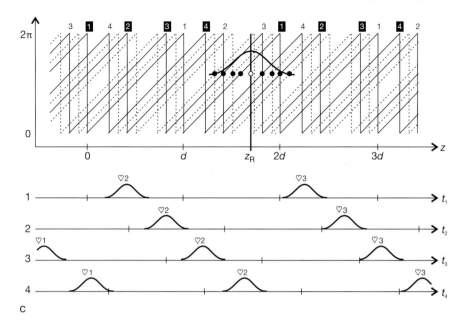

disadvantage is the fact that the slice sensitivity profile is not defined exactly. The 180°MCI algorithms that are labeled as 'multi-sectoral', 'biphasic', or similar approach in the manufacturers' implementations represent the method of choice, in particular when higher heart frequencies are given.

With the rotation times available today, it is still preferable with respect to image quality to select phases of relatively slow heart motion, i.e., primarily the diastolic phase. It is possible, nevertheless, to generate images for any arbitrary heart phase by continuously shifting the selected ECG interval. Multi-planar and three-dimensional (3D) display of the heart in good quality can then be obtained for successive heart phases, providing the possibility for true 4D imaging of the heart. Examples are given in Figure 3 for a low and a high heart frequency. Systolic images are shown in the upper row for both cases, diastolic images are shown in the center row, and MPRs for diastole are shown in the bottom row. It is understood that no phase can be assigned to the standard reconstruction 180°MLI (multislice linear interpolation). Apparently, the special interpolation algorithm 180°MCI offers significant improvements with respect to temporal resolution, since only relatively short sections of the R-R interval are used. Depending on the relation of heart frequency and rotation frequency, effective scan times of less than 100 ms can be reached.

Respective results are quite impressive. It is difficult, however, to determine how sharp and how reliable such displays are for heart phases associated with fast motion. The clinical examples only allow a qualitative and subjective assessment. Simulations and subjective impressions have to be confirmed objectively by measurements. The quality control tools discussed in the next section will help to do so and to determine the optimal approach in cardiac imaging.

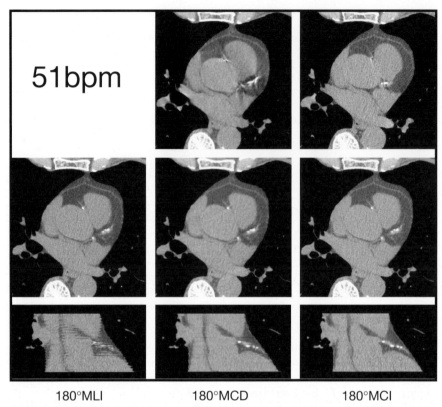

180°MLI   180°MCD   180°MCI

Fig. 3a, b. Comparison of results for standard reconstructions [180°MLI (multislice linear interpolation), *left*] and for electrocardiogram-correlated image reconstruction. [180°MCD (multislice cardio delta), *center*; 180°MCI (multislice cardio interpolation), *right*]. A 51 bpm, b 95 bpm superior performance is exhibited by 180 MCI, especially for higher heart rates

Quality Assurance for Cardiac CT Imaging

It is generally expected that the heart can be imaged well if its structures do not move significantly during the time of the scan or, for retrospective approaches, during the effective scan time. For rotation times of 500 ms and for low heart frequencies, this assumption is valid to a high degree for the diastolic phase, where phases of relatively little motion are given for 250 ms or more in many cases. For higher heart frequencies and for other motion phases of the heart, this assumption no longer holds true. Scan times of less than 50 ms would be required to image the heart in all phases of motion without any influence of motion [6]. Consequently, imaging results may vary and special performance tests and quality assurance (QA) tools should be provided for cardiac CT.

Performance tests are needed to compare the different scanners, scan, and reconstruction protocols; QA and calibration tools are needed most for coronary calcium scoring, a quantitative CT application. Such tests must be suitable for conventional CT, and EBCT, and single- and multislice acquisition in spiral

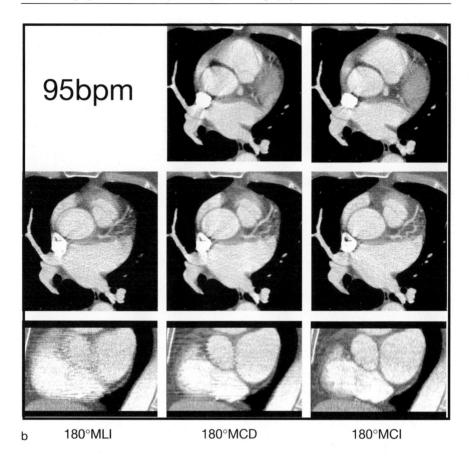

95bpm

b   180°MLI   180°MCD   180°MCI

mode with different retrospective ECG-correlated reconstructions. Performance tests for cardiac CT must only supplement the tests established generally for acceptance and constancy testing. Primarily, we aim at measurements of spatial resolution and calcium quantification for moving objects. Spatial resolution measurements are straightforward to a high degree when respective setups are available; a calibration for calcium scoring is more difficult to achieve since different sizes, shapes, and concentrations of calcified plaque may have to be taken into account.

Approaches for meeting the above demands are available. Figure 4a shows a QA phantom and respective calibration inserts which have been developed at the Institute of Medical Physics (IMP) in collaboration with Siemens Medical Systems, the phantom manufacturer (QRM GmbH, Möhrendorf, Germany) and users of the SOMATOM Volume Zoom. For the present, this only represents a proposal. A consensus regarding calibration standards and QA programs is still urgently needed.

A motion phantom setup is shown in Fig. 4b. Here, the calibration insert in the QA phantom is replaced by a water tank. A PC-controlled robot moves arbitrary

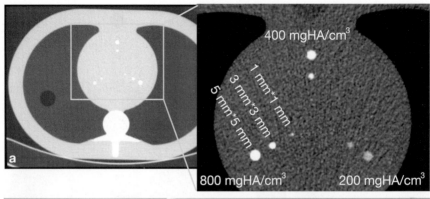

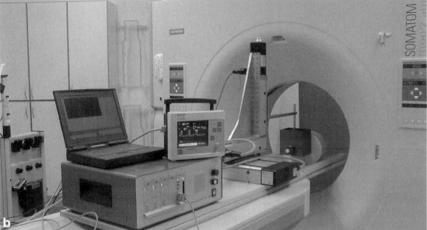

Fig. 4a–c. Quality control for coronary calcium measurements. An anthropomorphic thorax phantom with replaceable calibration inserts (**a**) for static calibration and a motion phantom (**b**) for dynamic studies enable the objective evaluation and comparison of different approaches (**c**)

small resolution tests or calcium inserts on freely programmable 3D paths at arbitrary frequencies, typically corresponding to between 30 bpm and 150 bpm. This allows for an easy comparison of results obtained with different approaches in a reproducible fashion. Figure 4c shows images obtained with the standard reconstruction 180°MLI and with the cardiac algorithms 180°MCD and 180°MCI at 90 bpm. The best performance is provided with 180°MCI. The reproducibility of the Agatston score [7] for coronary calcium was assessed for a 3 mm calcium cylinder with 400 mg calcium hydroxyapatite (HA)/cm^3 at different heart rates (40–100 bpm in steps of 10 bpm) for EBCT and for the Volume Zoom. Reproducibility was found to be 16% for EBCT and 14% and 5%, respectively, with 180°MCD and 180°MCI on the SOMATOM Volume Zoom in this test.

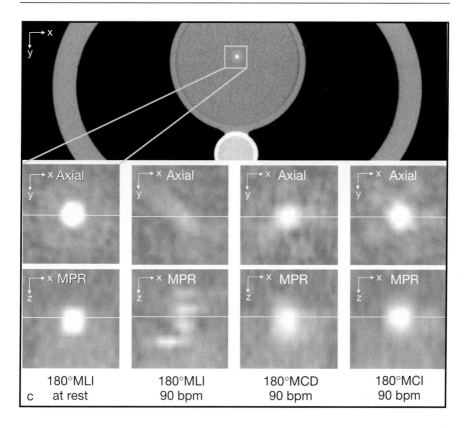

180°MLI	180°MLI	180°MCD	180°MCI
at rest	90 bpm	90 bpm	90 bpm

c

Conclusions

Effective scan times of below 100 ms can be achieved with subsecond multislice spiral CT. They have been verified for the SOMATOM Volume Zoom with 180°MCI in phantom experiments and patient scans. Even for tachycardic situations (>100 bpm) and irregular pulse frequencies, 180°MCI performed well. The freely programmable motion phantom in combination with the calibration phantom provides appropriate tools to compare results for different scan modalities.

In addition to imaging of the heart in general and to CT coronary angiography, phase-selective displays of the heart and measurement of coronary calcium content open a complete new field of application for CT. The high quality of results, as for example the display of a stenosis and of soft plaque (Fig. 5, left) here, demonstrated in direct comparison with conventional angiography (right), is astounding. Nevertheless, or even more so, quality control efforts are asked for.

The QA tools described above appear adequate; a consensus on test procedures and criteria is still necessary. This new field of application for CT is developing very rapidly. Long-term success will only be possible if the quality of the results, in particular reproducibility of calcium scoring results and comparability between different scanners, can be assured.

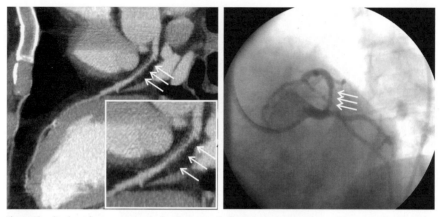

Fig. 5. The display of a stenosis and of soft plaque (*left*) in direct comparison with conventional angiography (*right*) demonstrates the high image quality and the high potential of subsecond multislice spiral CT for cardiac imaging

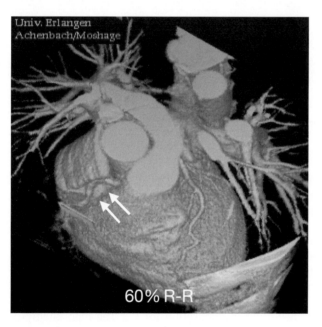

Fig. 6. Three-dimensional (3D) display of a heart which can also be viewed in animated fashion (see http://www.imp.uni-erlangen.de) for all heart cycles – the basis for functional 4D imaging of the heart. Even fast moving structures, such as the right coronary artery (*arrows*) in this example of shaded-surface display of the heart can be depicted without motion artifacts

Acknowledgements. All figures have been taken from a recent textbook on CT [8] with friendly permission of the publisher. We thank Drs. Achenbach, Baum, and Moshage of the University Hospital Erlangen for a very good cooperation and for providing the clinical images.

References

1. Kachelrieß M, Kalender WA, Karakaya M, Achenbach S, Nossen J, Moshage W, Bautz WA (1998) Imaging of the heart by ECG-oriented reconstruction from subsecond spiral CT scans. In: Glazer G and Krestin G (eds) Advances in CT IV. Springer, Heidelberg, Berlin, New York, pp 137–143
2. Bielak LF, Kaufmann RB, Moll PP, McCollough CH, Schwartz RS, Sheedy PF (1994) Small lesions in the heart identified at electron beam CT: calcification or noise? Radiology 192:631–636
3. Kachelrieß M, Kalender WA (1998) ECG-correlated image reconstruction from subsecond spiral ct scans of the heart. Medical Physics 25:2417–2431
4. Kachelriess M, Ulzheimer S, Kalender WA (2000) ECG-correlated image reconstruction from subsecond multi-slice spiral CT scans of the heart. Med Physics 27:1881–1902
5. Kachelriess M, Ulzheimer S, Kalender WA (2000) ECG-correlated imaging of the heart with subsecond multi-slice CT scans. IEEE transactions on medical imaging (in press)
6. Ritchie CJ, Godwin JD, Crawford CR, Stanford W, Anno H, Kim Y (1992) Minimum scan speeds for suppression of motion artifacts in CT. Radiology 185:37–42
7. Agatston A, Janowitz F, Hildner N, Zusmer M, Viamonte R, Detrano R (1990) Quantification of coronary artery calcium using ultrafast computed tomography. J Am Coll Cardiol 15:827–832
8. Kalender WA (2000) Computed tomography. Wiley and Sons, New York

The Potential of Cardio-Computed Tomography

Alexander v. Smekal

In order to determine the potential benefit of a new approach in cardiac imaging, it is important to define what we need to know, and how we can achieve this goal. There are two basic ways to look at the heart, a static and a dynamic one. With static visualization, morphological information can be obtained. Dynamic imaging also permits functional evaluation.

When speaking about cardiac morphology, coronary artery imaging is in everybody's mind. However, there is more: visualization of the heart and its chambers, imaging of the myocardium, pericardium, cardiac and para-cardiac masses, bypass grafts, and the relationship between the heart and the main thoracic vessels. The goal of imaging of cardiac function is to measure functional parameters of the heart, i.e. volume measurements of the chambers at different cardiac phases for calculation of different ratios, such as ejection fraction of the ventricles, myocardial thickening, myocardial mass, and myocardial perfusion and viability.

At present, various cardiac imaging modalities are in daily routine use. One can distinguish between modalities which are invasive or non-invasive, more or less risk-related, more or less comfortable for the patient, and more or less expensive. The currently performed methods are echocardiography and its invasive counterpart intravascular ultrasound, catheter angiography, nuclear medicine methods, such as single photon emission CT (SPECT) and positron emission tomography (PET), and magnetic resonance imaging.

Up to now, computed tomography (CT) was rarely used in cardiac imaging. The first attempts to utilize CT in cardiac imaging were made by Harell et al. [1] and by Lackner et al. [2]. This so-called stop action CT did not succeed due to technical limitations and high radiation exposure. The development of ultrafast or electron-beam CT (EBCT) [3] permitted data acquisition in 50 ms and 100 ms for one slice. EBCT is technically limited to partial scan acquisition (240°), but this technique opened the door to cardiac imaging. It became possible to synchronize data acquisition with the patient's electrocardiogram (ECG). The result of this synchronization is a decrease of cardiac motion artifacts and a real contiguous volume imaging at a specific time during the cardiac cycle (Fig. 1, 5).

With ECG-triggering the sequential data acquisition of a single slice is started at a specific time in the cardiac cycle, which is determined by the delay to the R-wave. This can be repeated in order to acquire a number of contiguous images during a patient's breathhold (Fig. 1). The volume of the scanned region is determined by scanner parameters, such as collimation, rotation time, and cycle time,

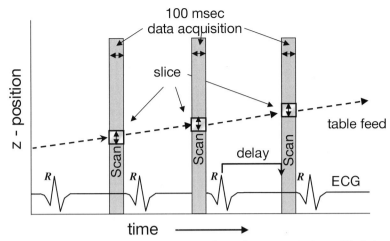

Fig. 1. ECG-triggering in EBCT. Due to the high cycle time of 0.8 s, data acquisition is possible during each RR interval in normo-frequent patients

and by patient parameters, such as heart rate and length of breathhold. ECG-triggering is a prospective synchronization method.

Using ECG-triggered EBCT and a cycle time of 0.8 s, imaging and measuring of coronary artery calcification became feasible. Some groups reported excellent results, but reproducibility was poor. The evaluation of coronary artery bypass graft patency became possible with high accuracy (Fig. 4a-b).

For detection and evaluation of coronary artery calcification, a non-contrast CT is required (Fig. 6). For almost all other purposes in cardio-CT, an intravenous injection of iodine contrast agent is needed.

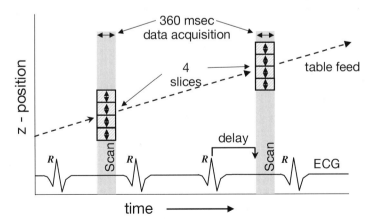

Fig. 2. ECG-triggering in multislice CT (four slices). The cycle time of 1.3 s permits data acquisition every second heart beat in normo-frequent patients. The acquisition of four slices at one time shortens study time with comparable parameters two- to threefold

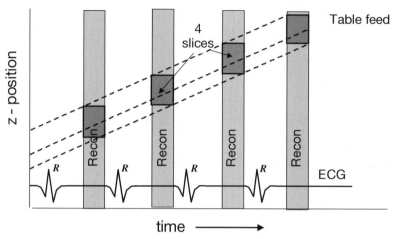

Fig. 3. ECG-gating permits visualization of multiple different time points during the cardiac cycle out of one spiral CT data set. This allows functional measurements

The advent of spiral CT technology [4] opened the way to fast data acquisition and volume imaging with conventional CT scanners. Sub-second rotation times enabled to visualize cardiac structures. However, volume imaging of the heart was greatly disturbed by motion artifacts due to multi-vectorial cardiac movements during the cardiac cycle.

ECG-triggering and sequential CT with partial scan imaging (240°) of these faster scanners permitted acquisition times of 500 ms per slice and thus much

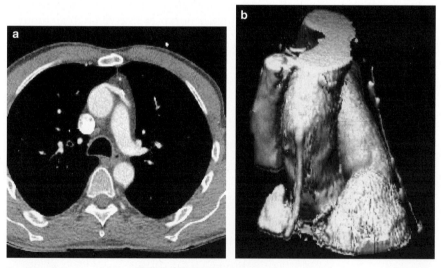

Fig. 4a, b. EBCT. **a** Axial slice with visualization of a venous coronary artery bypass graft (CABG) and its proximal anastomosis to the ascending aorta with adjacent clip. **b** Surface-shaded display with visualization of a venous CABG to the right coronary artery and an arterial graft of the left internal mammary artery (with adjacent clips) to the left anterior descending coronary artery

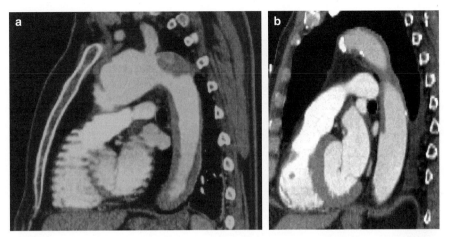

Fig. 5a, b. Effect of ECG-triggering on heart motion artifacts in multislice CT. **a** Non-ECG-triggered data acquisition with heart motion related disturbance of the visualization of the cardiac and vascular structures in sagittal multi-planar reconstruction (MPR). **b** ECG-triggered data acquisition with clear differentiation of the cardiac and vascular structures without heart motion artifacts in MPR. The mitral valve and the trabeculi can be clearly seen

better delineation of the cardiac structures. Due to contiguous slice positioning during one single breathhold, three dimensional visualization of cardiac structures became possible. On the other hand, the volume of the scanned region and the spatial resolution are limited by the ability of the patient to hold his breath.

The latest step in CT technology was the implementation of multislice imaging, i.e. simultaneous data acquisition of multiple slices during one gantry rotation. At this time, CT scanners can acquire two or four slices per rotation. At Siemens Medical Systems, this goes parallel with a decrease of the rotation time to 500 ms and to 350 ms partial scan (240°) time in sequential CT combined with a speed up in cycle time to 1.3 s. This permits thinner slicing to achieve nearly

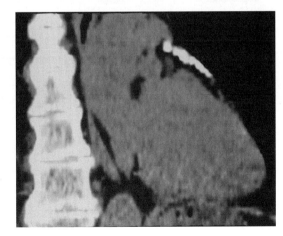

Fig. 6. Multi-planar reconstruction of a non-contrast enhanced ECG-triggered multislice CT data set for coronary artery calcification evaluation. The extensive calcification of the proximal left anterior descending coronary artery can be appreciated

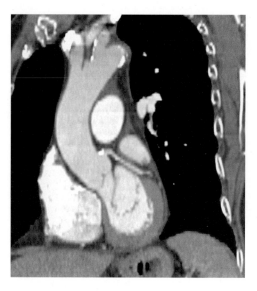

Fig. 7. Contrast-enhanced ECG-triggered multislice CT. Visualization of the proximal part of the left main and the left anterior descending coronary artery with calcification in the aorta and the coronary artery ostium. Clear delineation of the aortic and mitral valve

isotropic volume imaging. It is logical to implement ECG synchronization. ECG triggering is already in use in single-slice imaging and can be easily adapted to multi-slice imaging.

The acquisition time in multislice CT is more than four times faster than in single-slice CT and two to three times faster in EBCT, which yields an increase in spatial resolution of the volume of the imaged region (Fig. 2).

When comparing sequential EBCT and sequential multislice CT images at a given collimation, the signal to noise (S/N) ratio and the resolution of multislice CT is clearly better.

ECG gating has been used for years in magnetic resonance imaging. It consists of contiguous data acquisition with parallel registration of the patient's ECG.

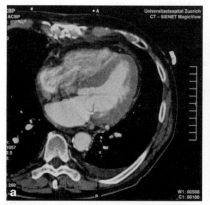
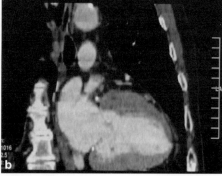

Fig. 8a, b. Multi-planar reconstruction of the heart based on classical echocardiographic planes from a contrast-enhanced ECG-triggered multislice CT data set. **a** Four chamber view, **b** two chamber view

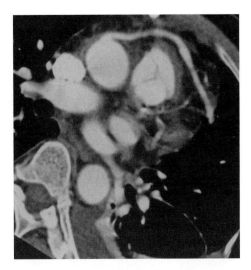

Fig. 9. Multi-planar reconstruction of a contrast-enhanced ECG-triggered data set to visualize coronary artery bypass patency. The course of a venous graft from its proximal anastomosis in direction to the left coronary artery can be seen. The pulmonary valve with its leaflets can be differentiated

Subsequent segmentation of the acquired data allows reordering and regrouping of certain data in concordance to the registered ECG for clear visualization of defined time points in the cardiac cycle (Fig. 3). This retrospective synchronization enables, for example, visualization of the myocardium of the same region in diastole and systole by using the same data set. The application of this method in CT opens a multitude of possibilities.

The advantage of ECG gating over ECG triggering is as follows: the data acquisition is independent from the patient's heart rate and visualization of the

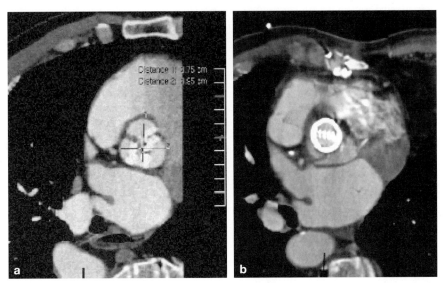

Fig. 10a, b. Aortic valve replacement. **a** Preoperative evaluation of morphology, size, and sclerosis of a aortic valve based on multi-planar reconstructions of a contrast-enhanced ECG-triggered multislice CT data set. **b** Postoperative control after aortic valve replacement

imaged region during multiple different times in the cardiac cycle is feasible. This permits functional evaluation. The disadvantage is the prolonged data post-processing and the associated higher radiation dose.

When considering all of the above mentioned points, one can summarize the value of cardio-CT in today's cardiac imaging:
1. Cardio-CT is multislice CT.
2. Multislice CT is superior to EBCT with regard to spatial resolution and S/N.
3. ECG triggering is a simple approach.
4. ECG gating is still complex with associated higher radiation dose.

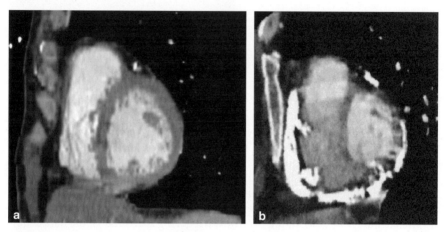

Fig. 11a, b. Comparison of a normal heart and a diseased heart with constrictive pericarditis. Contrast-enhanced ECG-triggered multislice CT data set. Multi-planar reconstruction of the short axis of the heart in end diastole. **a** Normal heart with normal size of the left and right ventricle. **b** Constrictive pericarditis with extensive pericardial calcifications and thinning of the left and right myocardium

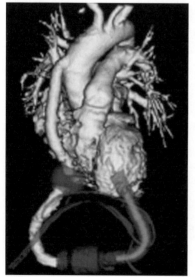

Fig. 12. Postoperative contrast-enhanced multislice CT and volume-rendered display of a patient with an implanted ventricular assist device (DeBakey VAD)

Therefore,
1. Cardio-CT is yet mainly visualization of morphology.
2. Cardio-CT is still limited by heart rate.

Cardio-CT is a simple, reliable, non-invasive, low risk, comfortable, and non-expensive cardiac imaging modality.

Today, cardio-CT permits evaluation of:
1. Cardiovascular morphology (Fig. 8 and Fig. 11)
2. Pre- and postoperative cardiovascular situation (Fig. 10 and Fig. 12)
3. Coronary artery calcification screening (Fig. 6)
4. Coronary angiography (characterization of coronary artery plaques) (Fig. 7)
5. Coronary artery bypass (Fig. 9)
6. Cardiac function to some extent

In the near future, ECG-gated multislice CT will be simplified and progress in technology will overcome some of today's limitations. For example, multi-phasic data sampling and new algorithms will allow data acquisition independently from the patient's heart rate. Imaging of cardiac function will be performed with isotropic spatial resolution. We witnessed an evolution from single-slice to four-slice CT imaging. However, will we really end with four-slice imaging ? How many slices will we experience with multislice CT?

References

1. Harell GS, Guthaner DF, Breimann RS, Mourehouse ChC, Seppi EJ, Marshall WH, Wexler L (1977) Stop-action cardiac computed tomography. Radiology 123:515–517
2. Lackner K, Simon H, Thun P (1979) Kardio-Computertomographie. Neue Möglichkeiten in der radiologischen nichtinvasiven Herzdiagnostik. Z Kardiol 68:667–675
3. Boyd DP, Lipton MJ (1983) Cardiac computed tomography. Proc IEEE 71:298–307
4. Kalender WA, Seissler W, Klotz E, Vock P (1990) Spiral volumetric CT with single-breath-hold technique, continuous transport, and continuous scanner rotation. Radiology 176:181–183

Coronary Atherosclerosis in Multislice Computed Tomography

Christoph R. Becker, Bernd M. Ohnesorge, U. Joseph Schoepf, Maximilian F. Reiser

Basic Principle of Coronary Computed Tomography Imaging

Cardiac imaging is a highly demanding application for any cross-sectional imaging modality. To virtually freeze cardiac motion and to avoid motion artifacts, high temporal resolution is needed. Many parts of the cardiac morphology, and especially the coronary arteries, represent small and complex three-dimensional (3D) structures that require high and at best sub-millimeter isotropic spatial resolution. For the last decade, computed tomography (CT) investigation of the heart was exclusively the domain of electron beam CT (EBCT). In these dedicated cardiac CT scanners, electrons are accelerated in a vacuum funnel and focused on four 210° tungsten target rings underneath the patient. X-ray radiation is emitted, passing through the patient, and is detected using two 240° detector rings above the patient. The design of these scanners was primarily chosen to allow for perfusion [17] and cine [12] imaging of the myocardium at eight levels, combined with a minimal exposure time of 50 ms per slice.

Morphological assessment of cardiac structures became possible with EBCT using a slice by slice acquisition and prospective electrocardiogram (ECG) triggering at 100 ms temporal resolution. To reduce cardiac motion and to scan the heart at a reproducible level, ECG triggering is essential. For prospective ECG triggering, which is currently being used for EBCT, the next RR interval (cardiac cycle: from R-wave to R-wave of the ECG) has to be estimated based on the median or mean of the last three to seven RR intervals in order to predict the mid-diastolic phase of the following RR interval. Scans acquired at mid diastole were found to have the least cardiac motion artifacts in most of the patients. Nevertheless, prospective ECG triggering is of limited use in patients with arrhythmia and is also affected by physiologic changes of the heart rate during a breath hold [18].

Principles of Coronary Multislice CT

In 1998, systems with four-slice detector arrays and a minimum rotation time of 500 ms that provide an eightfold performance relative to a 1-s rotation single-slice CT system were introduced. The combination of fast rotation time and multislice acquisition is particularly important for cardiac applications.

Using ECG-triggered sequential scanning, four slices can be acquired simultaneously with each prospectively ECG-triggered scan with a temporal resolution

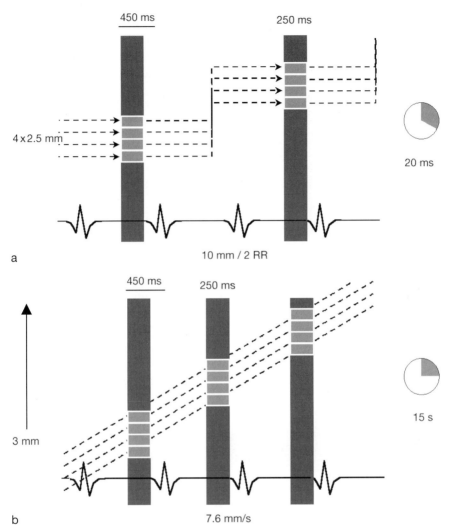

Fig. 1a–f. Scanning protocols for coronary screening multislice computed tomography (MSCT) with prospective electrocardiogram (ECG) triggering (**a**) and retrospective ECG gating (**b**). Retrospective ECG gating with MSCT allows for coronary angiography with 1.25 mm slice thickness (**c**). The currently available exposure time of 250 ms is sufficient for imaging the heart without motion artifacts up to a heart rate of 70 bpm (**d**). Optimized reconstruction algorithms reach minimum 125 ms exposure time (**e**), allowing the investigation of patients with higher heart rates (**f**)

of 250 ms using routine 500 ms rotation time and partial scan acquisition [15, 20]. Usually, the trigger delay is defined in a way that the scans are acquired during the mid-diastolic phase of the heart. The scan time to cover the whole heart is about 20 s with 2.5-mm slices (Fig. 1a). The acquisition with four adjacent slices may reduce the risk of slice overlap or gap that can occur with single-slice acquisition due to cardiac motion in the z-direction.

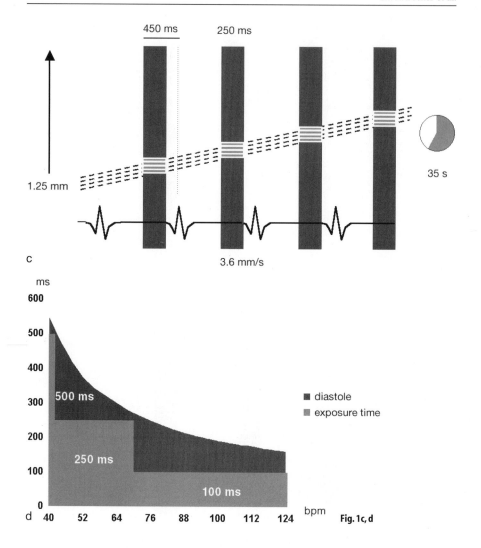

Fig. 1c, d

In addition, MSCT with the new technique of retrospective ECG gating is able to overcome the limitations of prospective ECG triggering with inconsistent heart phase scanning when arrhythmia is present. For this approach, slow table motion during spiral scanning and simultaneous acquisition of four slices and the digital ECG trace are employed to perform an oversampling of scan projections. This technique can either be used to investigate the heart in a shorter scan time (15 s) with the commonly used 3-mm slices (Fig. 1b) or still in a reasonable breath hold time (30–35 s), with a thinner slice thickness (1.25 mm; Fig. 1c) compared with single scan acquisition. In our department, the first protocol is currently used for detection and quantification of coronary calcium, whereas the second protocol is tailored to assess the changes of the coronary artery wall by contrast-enhanced CT angiography.

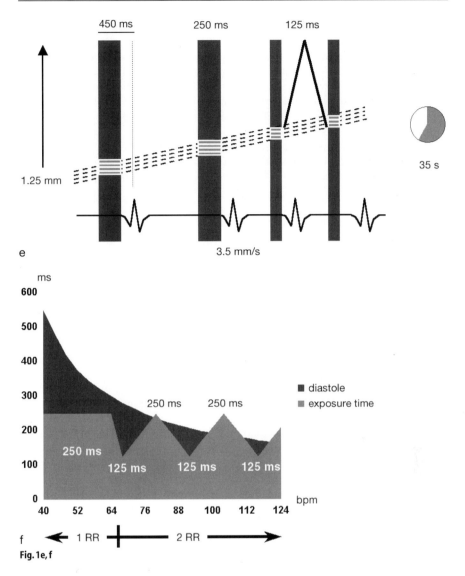

Fig. 1e, f

As data are acquired continuously during ECG-gated spiral scanning and a dedicated cardiac phase is targeted by means of retrospective selection of the appropriate data, X-ray radiation of the retrospective ECG spiral gating is higher than prospective ECG sequence triggering. However, with retrospective ECG gating, images can be reconstructed with small slice increment, thus improving the quality of 3D reconstruction and the reproducibility of a coronary calcium measurement, and at different cardiac phases.

Partial scan-based spiral algorithms that use 240° data segments in each cardiac cycle provide 250 ms temporal resolution [21, 22] with 500 ms rotation time, sufficient for a heart rate below 70 bpm (Fig. 1d). Dedicated spiral reconstruction algorithms that are optimized with regard to temporal resolution are available. Depending on the relation of rotation time and heart rate, the temporal resolution can be improved up to 125 ms by using data from two consecutive cardiac cycles for image reconstruction (Fig. 1e). Compromising on spatial resolution for up to 125 ms, temporal resolution can be avoided by performing this kind of algorithm for heart rates above a certain limit only (Fig. 1f). With this adaptive approach, no decrease of spiral pitch is needed and thus can be performed also with 1.25 mm slice thickness. Reconstruction algorithms can be extended to use data from more than two consecutive cardiac cycles to provide even higher temporal resolution (<100 ms). However, this very high temporal resolution can then only be achieved at the expense of spatial resolution (3 mm slices) [9, 14].

Detection and Quantification of Coronary Calcium

Unenhanced scans of the heart clearly display any calcifications of the coronary artery tree. As arterial calcifications almost always represent atherosclerosis, EBCT was shown to be the most sensitive tool to detect coronary atherosclerosis and is even superior to fluoroscopy [1] for this application. Primarily, detection of coronary calcifications has been used to determine the presence of coronary artery disease (CAD) in symptomatic patients with atypical chest pain [16]. Nevertheless, the value of detecting coronary calcifications alone is limited by age and gender, depending on the prevalence and extent of the coronary calcium plaque burden [13]. To overcome this limitation, quantitative assessment of coronary calcium was first introduced by Agatston et al. [1]. The amount of coronary calcium was semi-quantitatively determined using a scoring method based on a slice by slice analysis of EBCT images. The score was used to compare the amount of coronary calcium in patients with and without clinical CAD, showing a significant difference in the mean values of both groups. In addition, the scoring method also showed good correlation with the histomorphometric assessment of coronary calcium in cardiac specimens [19].

Recent studies found the determination of the calcium plaque volume to be superior to the established estimation of the calcium plaque burden with respect to reproducibility when using the Agatston scoring method [10]. With this improved 3D quantification algorithm, Callister et al. [11] were able to follow the regression of the volume of calcified plaques in patients treated with HMG-CoA reductase inhibitors (lipid-lowering drug).

It became evident that the detection and quantification of coronary calcium is also feasible with conventional CT scanners. Shemesh et al. performed measurements of coronary calcium with a dual helical CT scanner and found a high accuracy for the quantification of coronary calcium [24]. The direct comparison of score values from CT images derived from EBCT and conventional single detector CT scanners showed a very high correlation [4].

In contrast to EBCT, the slice thickness with MSCT is 2.5 mm and, therefore, the determination of the score either leads to a systematic error or has to be corrected using an additional factor in order to be comparable with score values derived from EBCT (3-mm slice thickness). However, the determination of the calcified plaque volume is independent from the slice thickness used and is therefore directly comparable between the two modalities [2].

The newest post-processing workstations determine the traditional 2D score and 3D-quantification algorithms, such as the volume, mass, and density of the coronary calcium plaque burden on the base of any CT modality. These semiautomatic workstations can help to increase inter-observer agreement. CT scanner calibration may help to determine absolute values for calcium mass or density for an accurate quantification and better comparison in the future. It is rather likely that the better reproducibility of volume, mass, and density measurements of the total plaque burden will replace the traditional score in the future [26].

As detection and quantification of coronary calcium may be mainly used as a screening tool in potentially healthy subjects, radiation exposure should be as low as possible. Indeed, for comparable image quality with EBCT and MSCT, the radiation exposure is similar with prospective ECG triggering [3]. Nevertheless, oversampling for retrospective ECG gating causes redundant X-ray radiation which, in most instances, is not used for reconstruction of the CT images.

A spiral acquisition allows reconstruction with a small slice increment and thus to improve the reproducibility of the calcium measurement. These advantages weigh most heavily in patients with a low amount of coronary calcium and in those with arrhythmia. In EBCT, the lack of reproducibility in these patients may be compensated for by performing two to three repeated scans of the cardiac volume, resulting in comparable radiation exposure similar to MSCT with retrospective gating. Nevertheless, the option of applying increased radiation with MSCT for decreasing image noise proved to be helpful for delineating minute calcified plaques against noise [8] even in obese patients (Fig. 2).

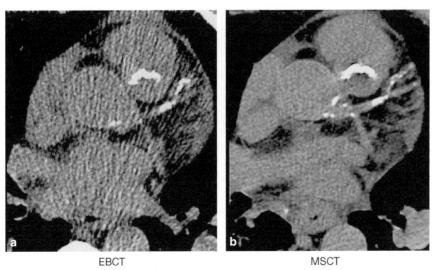

EBCT   MSCT

Fig. 2. Image comparison in a patient with calcifications in the left anterior descending coronary artery [electron beam computed tomography (EBCT) left, multislice computed tomography (MSCT) right]. With lower image noise, calcifications are displayed more clearly in the MSCT image

Coronary MSCT Angiography

Motion artifacts may be accepted to a certain degree for quantification of coronary calcium [6]. Nevertheless, for MSCT angiography (MSCTA), motion artifacts degrade image quality unacceptably for image analysis. Therefore, when contraindications have been ruled out, we regularly use β-blocker (50–100 mg metroprololtatrat) orally administered 1 h prior to the investigation to ensure sufficient image quality in patients with a heart rate significantly above 70 bpm.

In coronary CTA, we commonly observed different stages of coronary artery wall changes. These changes seem to be related to significant coronary artery disease by a certain pattern [5]. The apparently normal coronary artery wall is about 0.1 mm in size and therefore usually not visible in CTA images (Fig. 3a). Early atherosclerotic changes of coronary arteries may consist of calcified and non-calcified components. In these cases, the small calcifications seem to be the "tip of the iceberg", where the entire extent of coronary atherosclerosis is "under the surface" and becomes visible after contrast injection only (Fig. 3b). These non-calcified plaques are not well defined and tend not to be the site of significant CAD. Extensive coronary artery calcifications without any non-calcified plaque are also unlikely the location for significant CAD (Fig. 3c). Complex atherosclerotic changes may appear as clots of calcified and non-calcified plaques and seem to be related more often to significant CAD (Fig. 3d). Nevertheless, the most severe findings of coronary atherosclerosis reveal purely non-calcified plaques [7] that may either cause severe stenoses or may be prone to rupture (Fig. 3e). The final stage may be the thrombotic occlusion with enlargement of the coronary vessel filled with low attenuation material, surrounded by a highly attenuated coronary artery wall (Fig. 3f).

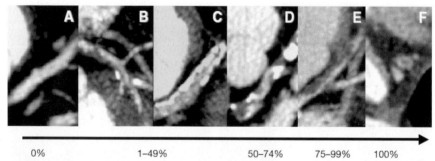

0%   1–49%   50–74%   75–99%   100%

Fig. 3a–f. Summary of different stages of coronary artery wall changes as seen using computed tomography (CT). These stages can be correlated with certain degrees of coronary artery stenoses. Calcifications tend to signal a minor degree of luminar narrowing, whereas humps of non-calcified plaques indicate significant coronary artery stenoses. The apparently normal coronary artery wall is about 0.100 μm in size and therefore usually not visible (**A**). Small calcifications seem to be the "tip of the iceberg", where the entire extent of coronary atherosclerosis is "under the surface" and becomes visible after contrast injection only (**B**). Extensive coronary artery calcifications without any non-calcified plaque are unlikely the location for significant coronary artery disease (CAD; **C**). Complex atherosclerotic changes may appear as clots of calcified and non-calcified plaques (**D**). Most severe findings of coronary atherosclerosis reveal purely non-calcified plaques (**E**). The final stage may be the thrombotic occlusion with enlargement of the coronary vessel filled with low attenuation material, surrounded by a highly attenuated coronary artery wall (**F**)

MSCTA Compared with Intravascular Ultrasound

The findings of MSCTA may best be correlated with intravascular ultrasound (IVUS). Currently, the most commonly used IVUS is performed with a 30 MHz transducer, allowing the determination of at least three different categories of coronary atherosclerosis. These three categories depend on the echogeneity of the atherosclerotic changes compared with the adventitia. The changes seen in IVUS may be either less dense, equally dense, or denser than the adventitia.

Direct comparison between MSCTA and IVUS confirms that non-calcified plaques in MSCTA correspond to soft tissue material on IVUS and, therefore, may consist of either fibrotic or lipid-rich plaques or even mixed plaques in the coronary artery wall. Other sites with heavy calcification on MSCTA correspond to areas which obviously consist of dense material on IVUS accompanied by a shadow, and thus may be identified as vessel calcification (Fig. 4). Again, soft tissue plaques tend to obstruct the lumen of the coronary vessel, whereas extensive calcified coronary artery vessels are remodeled and therefore non-obstructive.

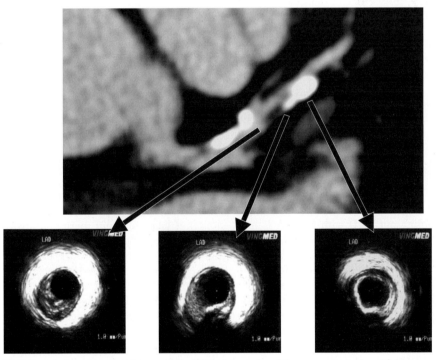

Fig. 4. Correlation of computed tomography (CT) angiography of the coronary arteries with intravascular ultrasound illustrates the ability of multislice CT to demonstrate calcified and non-calcified coronary plaques

Clinical Use and Future Aspects

As the detection and quantification of coronary calcium with EBCT corresponds well to the measurement with conventional (single, dual, and multi-row detector) CT, the current discussion on the clinical value of coronary screening can be extended to any of the CT modalities currently in use for this purpose. The most crucial question concerning coronary calcifications is whether future cardiac events in asymptomatic patients with cardiovascular risk factors can be predicted based on CT measurements. Detection of coronary calcium alone would lead to an overestimation of the risk of future coronary events, especially in young asymptomatic subjects [25].

In a meta-analysis, based on the current literature performed by O'Malley et al. [23], a summary risk ratio of 8.7:1 (95% confidence interval 2.7–28.1) was found for a combined outcome (nonfatal myocardial infarction, death, or revascularization). In contrast to this, the total risk ratio for hard events only (myocardial infarction or death) was significantly lower (4.2:1; 95% confidence interval 1.6–11.3) than for the combined risk. However, there was significant heterogeneity in the studies' quality and patient populations. Therefore, the authors concluded that there is still a need for larger and longer prospective cohort studies of a non-self-referred screening population, particularly of younger ages than in previous studies. In addition, it needs to be determined whether the observed association with hard outcomes is strong enough to make screening with CT superior or more cost-effective than standard risk factor assessment.

As already stated, the potential role of screening for coronary calcifications to determine the risk for future cardiac events needs to be evaluated more thoroughly by means of prospective cohort studies and adequate methods for quantification as described above. But even with the absolute determination of coronary calcium, further improvement in the clinical value or additional clinical applications for the detection and quantification of coronary calcifications is not to be expected.

In contrast to this, the potential role of MSCTA for patient investigations became most obvious in recent months. Once the negative predictive value for ruling out CAD with MSCTA is high enough, it helps to avoid mere diagnostic cardiac catheterizations in those patients with unspecific chest complaints and in those where non-invasive stress testing remains unspecific. Most probably, women may benefit most from ruling out CAD by means of MSCTA because of the lack of a specific stress test in this patient group. Even young patients without symptoms but with a very high risk of cardiovascular disease may benefit from MSCTA, which allows the demonstration of the presence or absence of the earliest signs of coronary atherosclerosis.

In addition, the resolution of MSCTA will prove to be sufficient to determine the patency of coronary vessels of coronary stents (Fig. 5) and bypass grafts (Fig. 6) after balloon angioplasty. We use this technique also to reliably detect thrombotic material within the heart chambers (Fig. 7) and infarcted myocardium (Fig. 8).

Shorter exposure times are desirable to dismiss the necessity for patient preparation. In MSCT with retrospective ECG gating, improved temporal resolution

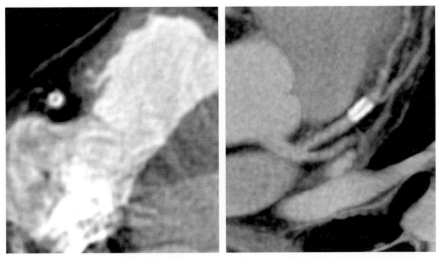

Fig. 5. Coronary stents look like circular calcifications or "railway tracks" depending on their location

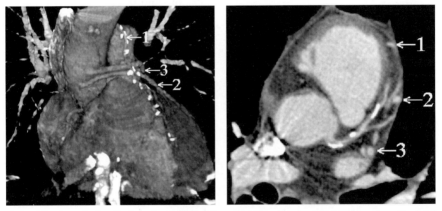

Fig. 6. Volume rendering displays the course of the venous (2+3) and arterial (1) bypass grafts. Axial slice clearly demonstrates the patency of the arterial (LIMA→LAD) and venous (ACVB→2.Dx, ACVB→RCx) grafts. LIMA, left anterior mammarian artery; LAD left anterior descending coronary artery; ACVB, aorto coronary venous bypass; Dx, diagnonal branch; RCx, circumflex coronary artery)

can be realized by alternative reconstruction algorithms, sampling data from more than one RR interval. This way, however, the oversampling rate will increase by slowing the table speed, while spatial resolution will decrease, at least with the current detector design. The use of a multi-detector design with more and thinner slices and faster gantry rotation will certainly overcome this problem.

Guidance by distinct evaluation of the time density curve of a test bolus may help to determine the optimal protocol for contrast administration. In addition, it may allow for a significantly better use of contrast media and for a reduction in

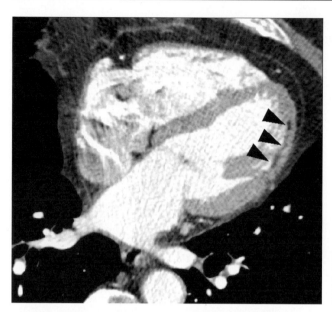

Fig. 7. Hypodense area in the lateral wall reflecting a myocardial infarction below the papillarian muscle

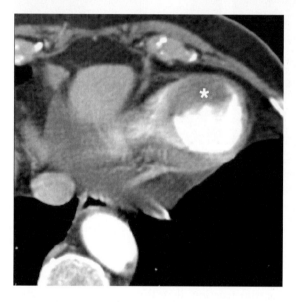

Fig. 8. Left ventricular aneurysm in a female patient after anterior wall myocardial infarction. The aneurysm is partly filled with a thrombus (*)

the amount of contrast media to about 60–80 ml. Morphology of the coronary artery may often not allow for determination of the relevancy of stenosis. Therefore, an investigation of the functional cardiac parameters is mandatory and may be obtained from a retrospective ECG-gated acquisition. Currently, post-processing software for functional evaluation of the cine reconstruction is not yet available.

Acknowledgements. The authors want to thank Andreas Knez, Alexander Leber, and Ralph Haberl from the Department of Internal Medicine–Cardiology, and Hendrik Treede from the Department of Cardiac Surgery for referring patients and for discussing the results. In addition, the authors want to thank Thomas Flohr from Siemens Medical Systems for supplying the newest MSCT technology. Finally the authors want to thank Cheng Hong from the Department of Clinical Radiology for assisting in the reconstruction of the CT images.

References

1. Agatston AS, Janowitz WR, Hildner FJ, Zusmer NR, Viamonte M, Detrano R (1990) Quantification of coronary artery calcium using ultrafast computed tomography. J Am Coll Cardiol 15:827–832
2. Becker C, Jakobs T, Knez A, Haberl R, Brüning R, Schöpf U, Reiser M (1998) Methoden zur Quantifizierung von Koronarkalk mit der Elektronenstrahl- und der konventionellen Computertomographie. Radiologe 38:1006–1011
3. Becker C, Schätzl M, Feist H, Bäuml A, Schöpf U, Michalski G, Lechel U, Hengge M, Brüning R, Reiser M (1999) Abschätzung der effektiven Dosis fuer Routineprotokolle beim konventionellen CT, Elektronstrahl-CT und bei der Koronarangiographie. Fortschr Röntgenstr 170:90–104
4. Becker C, Jakobs T, Aydemir S, Becker A, Knez A, Schöpf U, Brüning R, Haberl R, Reiser M (2000) Helical and single slice conventional versus electron beam CT for quantification of coronary artery calcification. AJR Am J Roentgenol 174:543–547
5. Becker C, Knez A, Leber A, Hong C, Treede H, Wildhirt S, Ohnesorge B, Flohr T, Schoepf U, Reiser M (2000) Erste Erfahrungen mit der Mehrzeilen-Detektor-Spiral-CT in der Diagnostik der Atherosklerose der Koronargefässe. Radiologe 40:118–122
6. Becker C, Knez A, Ohnesorge B, Schoepf U, Flohr T, Bruening R, Haberl R, Reiser M (2000) Visualisation and quantification of coronary calcifications with electron beam and spiral computed tomography. Eur Radiol 10:629–635
7. Becker C, Knez A, Ohnesorge B, Schoepf U, Reiser M (2000) Imaging of noncalcified coronary plaques using helical CT with retrospective ECG gating. AJR Am J Roentgenol 175:423–424
8. Bielak LF, Kaufmann RB, Moll PP, McCollough CH, Schwartz RS, Sheedy PF (1994) Small lesions in the heart identified at electron beam CT: calcification or noise? Radiology 192:631-636
9. Bruder H, Schaller S, Ohnesorge B, Mertelmeier T (1999) High temporal resolution volume heart imaging with multirow computed tomography. SPIE 3661:420–432
10. Callister T, Cooil B, Raya S, Lippolis N, Russo D, Raggi P (1998) Coronary artery disease: improved reproducibility of calcium scoring with an electron beam CT volumetric method. Radiology 208:807–814
11. Callister T, Raggi P, Cooli B, Lippolis N, Russo D (1998) Effect of HMG-CoA reductase inhibitors on coronary artery disease as assessed by electron-beam computed tomography. N Engl J Med 339:1972–1978
12. Himelman R, Abbott J, Lipton M, Schiller N (1988) Cine computed tomography compared with echocardiography in the evaluation of cardiac function in emphysema. Am J Cardiac Imaging 2:283–291
13. Janowitz W, Agatston A, Kaplan G, Viamonte M (1993) Differences in prevalence and extent of coronary artery calcium detected by ultrafast computed tomography in asymptomatic men and women. Am J Cardiol 72:247–254
14. Kachelries M and Kalender W (1998) Electrocardiogram-correlated image reconstruction from subsecond spiral computed tomography scans of the heart. Med Phys 25:2417–2431
15. Klingenbeck-Regn K, Schaller S, Flohr T, Ohnesorge B, Kopp A, Baum U (1999) Subsecond multislice computed tomography: basics and applications. Eur J Radiol 31:110–124
16. Laudon D, Vukov L, Breen J, Rumberger J, Wollan P, Sheedy P (1999) Use of electron-beam computed tomography in the evaluation of chest pain patients in the emergency department. Ann Emerg Med 33:15–21
17. Lipton MJ and Holt WW (1991) Computed tomography for patient management in coronary artery disease. Circulation 84:172–180
18. Mao S, Oudiz R, Bakhsheshi H, Wang S, Brundage B (1996) Variation of heart rate and electrocardiograph trigger interval during ultrafast computed tomography. Am J Cardiac Imaging 10:239–243

19. Mautner GC, Mautner SL, Froehlich J, Feuerstein IM, Proschan MA, Roberts WC, Doppman JL (1994) Coronary artery calcification: assessment with electron beam CT and histomorphometric correlation. Radiology 192:619–623

20. Ohnesorge B, Flohr T, Schaller S, Klingenbeck-Regn K, Becker C, Schöpf U, Brüning R, Reiser M (1999) Technische Grundlagen und Anwendungen der Mehrschicht-CT. Radiologe 39:923–931

21. Ohnesorge B, Flohr T, Becker C, Knez A, Kopp A, Fukuda K, Reiser M (2000) Herzbildgebung mit schneller, retrospektiv EKG-synchronisierter Mehrschichtspiral CT. Radiologe 40:111–117

22. Ohnesorge B, Flohr T, Becker C, Kopp A, Knez A, Baum U, Klingenbeck-Regn K, Reiser M (2000) Cardiac imaging with ECG-gated multi-slice spiral CT – initial experience. Radiology 217:(in press)

23. O'Malley P, Taylor A, Jackson J, Doherty T, Detrano R (2000) Prognostic value of coronary electron-beam computed tomography for coronary heart disease events in asymptomatic populations. Am J Cardiol 85:945–948

24. Shemesh J, Apter S, Rozenman J, Lusky A, Rath S, Itzchak Y, Motro M (1995) Calcification of coronary arteries: detection and quantification with double-helix CT. Radiology 197:779–783

25. Wexler L, Brundage B, Crouse J, Detrano R, Fuster V, Maddahi J, Rumberger J, Stanford W, White R, Taubert K (1996) Coronary artery calcification: pathophysiology, epidemiology, imaging methods, and clinical implications. A statement for health professionals from the American Heart Association. Circulation 94:1175–1192

26. Yoon HC, Greaser LE, Mather R, Sinha S, McNitt Gray MF, Goldin JG (1997) Coronary artery calcium: alternate methods for accurate and reproducible quantitation. Acad Radiol 4:666–673

Coronary Computed Tomography Angiography Using Multislice Computed Tomography: Pitfalls and Potential

Malte L. Bahner, J. M. Boese

When we first applied retrospective gating on the singleslice scanner Siemens SOMATOM Plus 4 for improvement of cardiac imaging in 1997, we did not expect the tremendous possibilities of this new, fast evolving tool for spiral computed tomography (CT). By now, we have greatly enhanced our thoughts on possible clinical settings and indications for cardiac spiral CT, and learned about some possible inherent new artifacts not known in standard CT.

With retrospective electrocardiogram (ECG) gating, the possible advantages of spiral CT over conventional CT can also be applied to imaging of the coronary arteries. In a first study, we evaluated the feasibility of this approach to improve imaging of coronary arteries with spiral CT.

We included 30 patients with indication for spiral CT of the thorax into this study. After approval by the institutional review board, written informed consent was obtained from each patient after the procedure was explained to its full extent. Imaging was performed with a SOMATOM Plus 4 singleslice scanner (Siemens AG, Forchheim, Germany). The imaging parameters included slice collimation 5 mm, rotation time 0.75 s, pitch 1.0, 120 kV, 150 mA, and standard adult body kernel (AB50). Intravenous contrast agent (Ultravist 300, Schering AG, Berlin, Germany) was administered via an indwelling forearm cannula according to the clinical question.

An ECG of each patient was acquired with a standard ECG monitor (Hellige, Sweden). The ECG signal was digitized via an analog–digital converter (ADC) in a PC. The 'X-ray ON' signal was obtained from the gantry and also digitized with the same ADC. Both signals were stored together and analyzed with a self-written software for determination of reconstruction start points.

Image reconstruction was performed on the CT scanner in two ways: standard continuous slim interpolation with an increment of 5 mm, and ECG-gated quick scan reconstructions with a temporal resolution of 500 ms. Reconstruction start points of ECG-gated images were calculated 500 ms before the next R wave in order to have the highest probability of including projections acquired during diastole. The resulting increment depended on the heart rate of each patient.

Images were filmed and placed to an alternator. One series, either non-gated or ECG-gated images, were randomly placed on the upper tray, while the other one covered the lower tray. No visible data gave hint to the used reconstruction method. Evaluation was performed by two consensus readers. Different anatomical structures were evaluated whether they were identical with both methods or the images of the upper tray were better or worse than the images on the lower

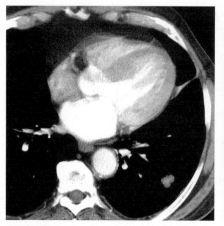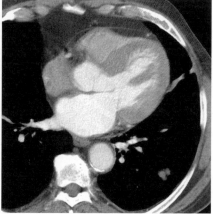

Fig. 1. Severe movement artifacts in the non-gated image (*left*) disables clear visualization of all coronary arteries. The right coronary artery (RCA) especially demonstrates this typical finding. In the gated image (*right*), the reduction of motion leads to a clear depiction of all three coronary arteries and the myocardium and pericardium

tray. If a structure was not visible in both methods, it was excluded from evaluation. For statistical analysis a Dixon and Mood statistics was performed.

Reconstruction of ECG-gated quick scan images was possible in all patients. Evaluation of the ECG and reconstruction of the ECG-gated images took approximately 5 min. ECG gating improved the quality of appearance for all evaluated coronary arteries: the left main stem, the proximal and distal left anterior descending artery (LAD), the proximal and distal left circumflex artery (LCX), and the proximal and distal right coronary artery (RCA). The ascending aorta, the aortic valve, the left ventricular wall, and the pericardium were also significantly better depicted. The mitral valve showed no statistically different appearance. ECG-gated images are shown in comparison with non-gated images of corresponding positions in Figures 1, 2.

The two limiting factors for this technique are scanning time and image acquisition time. While the diastole covers approximately two-thirds of the heart cycle, an acquisition time of 500 ms is only short enough if the heart rate is sufficiently low. In addition, the pitch for spiral scanning needs to be adapted to the heart rate of the individual patient [1]. Thus, scanning time would be approximately 60 s on the singleslice SOMATOM Plus 4 with 750 ms rotation time if the slice collimation was reduced to 2 mm.

The introduction of the multislice CT scanner SOMATOM Volume Zoom with simultaneous acquisition of four slices per rotation and an increased rotation speed of 500 ms for 360° brought important improvements for cardiac CT scanning. Combined with retrospective cardiac gating, it offers the chance for non-invasive imaging of cardiac morphology, coronary and valvular calcifications, and the coronary vessels using CT angiography (CTA). In addition, with further improved temporal resolution to calculate images during systole, it is possible to acquire functional data of the heart and the aorta in a 'one-stop shop' approach. Nevertheless, this technique is more complicated than conventional CT. In the

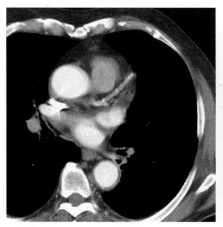 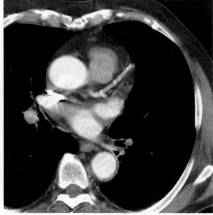

Fig. 2. The non-gated image (*left*) only has a small amount of movement artifacts. Nevertheless, the gate image (*right*) depicts the morphology of the aorta, the left anterior descending artery (LAD), and its subtle calcifications more clearly

following, an overview of the most common problems and artifacts of cardiac spiral CT is given.

Calcifications Obscuring Vessel Lumen

In regions with severe calcifications of the vessel wall, the residual small lumen of the artery might be hard to evaluate due to the neighboring high contrast of the calcium deposition (Fig. 3). This might be a blooming effect of the high density of the severely calcified plaque. This will potentially lead to an overestimation of the grade of an underlying stenosis.

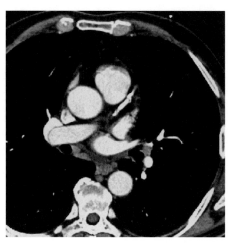

Fig. 3. An underlying stenosis can only be anticipated in this severely calcified left anterior descending artery (LAD). The actual grade of stenosis is overestimated on this image alone due to blooming effects of the high attenuation calcium

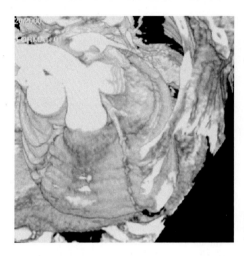

Fig. 4. Phase shift artifact of the left anterior descending artery (LAD) in volume-rendered three-dimensional display

Phase Shift Artifact

Another problem of cardiac CT with retrospective gating is the variability of cardiac rhythm. On a four-detector system, every fourth slice is acquired within a different cardiac cycle. Thus, variations between gating time and heart phase lead to a shift between adjacent slices. This so-called phase shift artifact especially occurs in patients with severely irregular heart rhythm. Its major consequence is that it might jeopardize three-dimensional (3D) display (Fig. 4). For the pure diagnosis of the grade of stenosis, this is most probably not of importance, because the transaxial images are not hampered by this artifact. Nevertheless, 3D display might prove to be essential for diagnosing and communicating results from CTA of the coronary arteries. Further work in understanding the physical properties of this artifact might help to reduce this problem in the future.

Limited Contrast Enhancement Distal to a High-Grade Stenosis

Another difficulty with coronary CTA is vascular opacification of small, distal segments when high-grade stenoses are present (Fig. 5). This mainly depends on the reduced flow of contrast agent through the relevant stenosis. In these cases, an increased opacification of the vessels, e.g., by increasing the flow rate or the iodine concentration, might lead to a better opacification even of small distal vessels. This will, however, result in high-density artifacts at the level of the atrium. Ongoing studies, especially in patient populations with severe CAD, will provide the data needed for designing adequate contrast injection protocols.

Motion Artifacts

Furthermore, limited temporal resolution is still a problem. Even with a time window of 250 ms, motion artifacts can hamper the visualization of structures

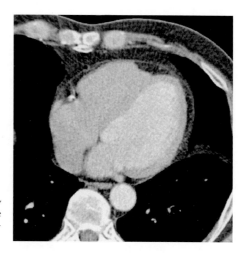

Fig. 5. The left anterior descending artery (LAD) is only depictable as a small structure within the pericardial fat with no visible contrast enhancement

moving at high velocities, e.g., the RCA. Algorithms that use data from more than one cardiac cycle for reconstruction of an image can improve temporal resolution, however, at the expense of the slice profile. This might especially be an advantage in applications, such as functional imaging of the ventricle movement,

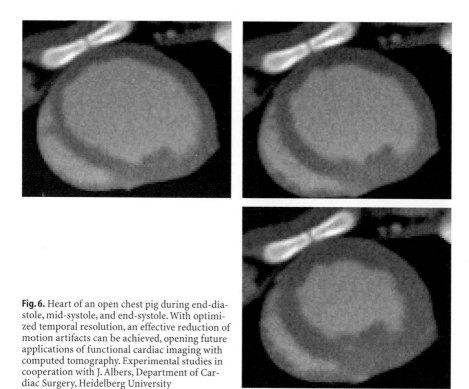

Fig. 6. Heart of an open chest pig during end-diastole, mid-systole, and end-systole. With optimized temporal resolution, an effective reduction of motion artifacts can be achieved, opening future applications of functional cardiac imaging with computed tomography. Experimental studies in cooperation with J. Albers, Department of Cardiac Surgery, Heidelberg University

where high z-resolution is not as crucial as in coronary CTA. In coronary angio-graphy, especially when combined with virtual endoscopy, high spatial resolution is essential. Thus, the increase in temporal resolution might not compensate for the loss in z-resolution. A compromise between temporal resolution and slice profile has to be found. More pitfalls not known yet will evolve with increased use of this new technique, while the knowledge in dealing with these artifacts and errors will also increase.

The potential of cardiac spiral CT is hard to imagine at the moment. Clear advantages over other existing techniques, such as electron beam CT are shown by other authors in this book. As a non-invasive method, it offers the possibility for an individualized risk assessment of CAD. This could, in the long run, lead to an improvement in treatment of patients at risk for cardiac events and in re-ducing overall costs of cardiac disease. Due to the good spatial resolution, CT might also play a role as a problem solver for altered cardiac morphology, when cardiac catheterization, echocardiography, and magnetic resonance (MR) imaging do not supply conclusive results. There might also be a role for CT in detailed operation planning of coronary bypass surgeries. Ongoing studies are evaluating this and show very promising preliminary results at this time.

As mentioned above, a 'one-stop shop' approach for assessment of cardiac morphology, cardiac and vascular pathology, and cardiac function is within reach. An important issue on this way is the validation of the different functional

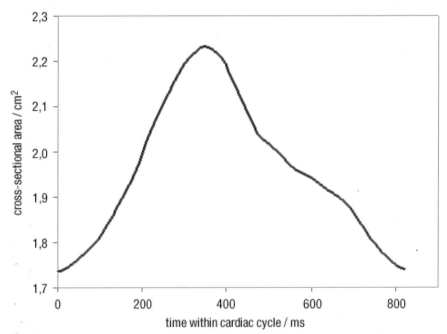

Fig. 7. Area of the aorta over the time during one heart cycle. This curve was calculated from electro-cardiogram (ECG)-gated computed tomography images in a pig in vivo using optimized temporal resolution

imaging methods against established standards. Preliminary, not yet published results from an ongoing experimental study with open chest pigs show a very good correlation of invasively measured stroke volumes with those calculated from spiral CT scans with retrospective ECG gating and improved temporal resolution by oversampling. The calculated data sets offer an isotropic resolution of 0.5 mm in combination with a temporal resolution in the range of 100–150 ms. At the moment, there is no other imaging modality offering this combination of imaging parameters in combination with the known short scanning time of spiral CT. This is especially important when imaging severely sick cardiac patients, where tight online surveillance is crucial.

Future tasks of functional imaging of the cardiovascular system will look at wall movement disorders, myocardial perfusion, and functional assessment of the ascending and descending aorta. These tasks are, at the moment, at a very experimental stage, but will be available within the next years. Examples of cardiac wall movement in an experimental pig model imaged during different phases of the heart cycle are shown in Figure 6. Figure 7 displays the movement of the aortic wall over time, correlating with aortic compliance, giving information on the post-cardiac vascular system. The combination of these different imaging tasks, including cardiac and cardiovascular morphology and pathology and different aspects of cardiac function, will offer a tremendous potential available on a broad clinical basis for the advantage of our patients. Nevertheless, future study will have to prove the clinical impact of cardiac spiral CT on the outcome of cardiovascular disease.

References

1. Bahner ML, Boese JM, Wallschlaeger H, van Kaick G (1999) Spiral-CT des Herzens mit retrospektivem EKG-Gating. Elektromedica 67:37–41

Cardiac Multislice Computed Tomography: Screening and Diagnosis of Chronic Heart Disease

Multislice Computed Tomography for Calcium Scoring, Computed Tomography Angiography of the Coronary Arteries, and Cardiac Functional Analysis

ANDREAS F. KOPP, STEPHEN SCHRÖDER, AXEL KÜTTNER, CHRISTIAN GEORG, BERND OHNESORGE, CLAUS D. CLAUSSEN

Coronary artery disease (CAD) is the leading killer in Europe and the United States. CAD accounted for almost 600,000 deaths in Europe in 1998. Although many patients initially present with symptoms, about half of all patients have no symptoms before their sudden death. Thus, a screening test for CAD might help stratify coronary risk in asymptomatic adults. Since its introduction in 1983, electron beam computed tomography scanning (EBCT) has been proposed as a means of coronary calcium assessment for screening. However, direct visualization of the epicardial coronary arteries is necessary to establish the presence and focal severity of lumen disease. Selective coronary angiography is the only clinical method to accurately visualize and quantify coronary artery anatomy in vivo. This method provides exceptional spatial resolution and a general road map of the coronary system. More than one million diagnostic catheterizations are performed in the United States each year. Selective coronary angiography is expensive and requires at least a brief hospital stay and a period of observation for several hours after the procedure. A convenient noninvasive and safe means to perform coronary angiography clearly would be of clinical benefit. Promising results have been reported for EBCT with a decent sensitivity and specificity in the detection of coronary artery stenoses [12, 16]. A major caveat of this method is, however, the high incidence of motion artifacts, leading to uninterpretable images [1, 4]. This limitation might now be overcome by the emergence of superfast multislice CT (MSCT) technology with spiral scanning at high temporal (125 ms) and superior spatial (10 lp/cm) resolution [11].

Data Acquisition with MSCT

Multislice cardiac imaging can be done using two basic modes of operation for image acquisition: prospective triggering and retrospective gating. Prospective triggering is used for sequential imaging. Compared with single slice CT and EBCT, the major advantage of MSCT is the simultaneous acquisition of four slices per prospective ECG trigger. The scan time to cover heart anatomy over a 120 mm volume is reduced to about 15 s, i.e., well within a single breath hold (the exact time depends on the heart rate). A sample protocol on the Siemens SOMATOM Volume Zoom for sequential cardiac CT is: 4x2.5 mm collimation, 500 ms rotation, 250 ms temporal resolution, a cycle time of 1.5 s (the actual value depends on heart rate), and z-coverage of 120 mm in 18 s [7].

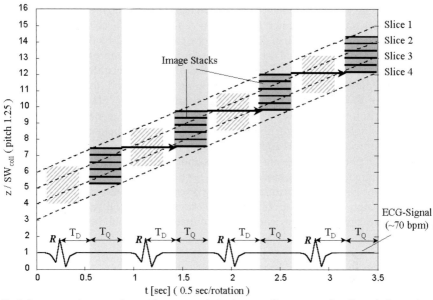

Fig. 1. Reconstruction procedure with retrospectively electrocardiogram-gated 4-slice spiral scanning

Retrospective gating is needed for spiral scanning. ECG gating can be performed with a "relative" or "absolute" approach. In a "relative" ECG-gating approach, the time delay is determined for each heart cycle individually as a certain fraction of the RR-interval. For "absolute" gating reconstruction, data is picked starting with a fixed time delay after a R-peak ("absolute-delay") or at a fixed time interval before a R-peak ("absolute-reverse"). Retrospective ECG gating was observed to improve cardiac image quality relative to prospective ECG-triggering techniques due to overlapping image reconstruction and reduced sensitivity to cardiac arrhythmia [14]. With four-slice spiral scanning, it is now for the first time possible to cover the entire volume of the heart within reasonable scan times using the technique of retrospective gating. For continuous volume coverage without gaps, the table speed (pitch) is adapted to the minimum heart rate of an individual patient (Fig. 1).

Adaptive Image Reconstruction

The cardiac MSCT algorithm provides a continuous volume image of the heart with a temporal resolution equal to half the rotation time ($T_{rot}/2$) in the individual slices. With unchanged rotation time, the temporal resolution can be improved by using scan data from more than one heart cycle for reconstruction of an image ("segmented reconstruction"). The partial scan data set for reconstruction of one image then consists of M projection sectors from different heart cycles. Depending on the relation of rotation time and patient heart rate, a temporal resolution within the interval [$T_{rot}/2$, $T_{rot}/2$ M] (M equals number of used heart cycles) can be achieved. However, for a given heart rate, segmented reconstruction requires lower spiral pitch to maintain gap-less volume coverage. The resulting increase in scan time usually needs to be compensated by thicker slice-collimation and thus reduced spatial z-resolution. A compromise on spatial resolution can be avoided by extending the μMSCV algorithm to a heart rate adaptive segmented reconstruction algorithm μ ("ACV") and restriction to maximum use of M=2 sectors. For the ACV algorithm, two sectors (M=2) are used for reconstruction at heart rates above a certain limit only (e.g., 68 bpm). The conventional single-sector algorithm MSCV (M=1) is used below that limit. This adaptive approach provides appropriate temporal resolution $T_{rot}/2$ for imaging in the diastolic phase at moderate heart rates and higher temporal resolution up to $T_{rot}/4$ for higher heart rates without a need for decreased spiral pitch and reduced z-resolution. The ACV algorithm can easily be extended to the use of M>2 sectors to achieve high temporal resolution at the expense of spatial resolution for imaging in the systolic phase where compromises on spatial resolution may be acceptable.

Clinical Applications

Calcium Scoring

Current EBCT protocols are used for measuring coronary arterial calcification by acquiring a stack of contiguous 3-mm thick sections [2]. The calcium score, as originally proposed by Agatston, is determined on the basis of the product of the total area of a calcified plaque and an arbitrary scoring system for those pixels with an attenuation greater than 130 HU. Theoretically, this multi-section data set should give a clear representation of the amount of calcification in the major coronary arterial tree, yet high interscan variability up to 60% has impaired the ability to measure coronary arterial calcification precisely and repeatedly [3, 5, 6, 15]. Spiral MSCT holds promise to overcome this limitation: coupling the technique of retrospective gating with nearly isotropic volumetric imaging, the reliability of coronary calcium quantification, especially for small plaques, was found to significantly improve. Using ECG-gated volume coverage with spiral MSCT and overlapping image reconstruction (2.5 mm collimation, 1 mm increment), an interscan variability of approximately 5% can be achieved [13]. With the advent of MSCT with significantly reduced interstudy variability, we can now begin to define the effects of treatment regimens on coronary arterial calcification and to determine whether changes in coronary arterial calcification in individual patients have predictive value for future coronary events. If these differences in calcium score over time result in a difference in event rates, it is conceivable that serial measurements of calcium score using MSCT will provide a powerful and much needed predictive tool.

CT Coronary Angiography

The imaging protocol for MSCT angiography (MSCTA) of the coronary arteries is relatively straightforward. To establish the scan delay time, a test bolus of 15 ml contrast medium and 20 ml saline chaser bolus is used. The circulation time is determined by measurements of CT density values in the ascending aorta. Imaging commences at the circulation time plus 3 s. A bolus of 120 ml nonionic contrast (370 mgI/ml) is injected trough an 18-gauge catheter into an antecubital vein at 4 ml/s followed by a 50 ml saline chaser bolus [10]. The scan protocol for the CTA per se is a spiral scan using 4x1 mm collimation (resulting in 1.25 mm slice width), 500 ms rotation time (with ACV up to 125 ms temporal resolution), 120 kV, 300 mA, and 0.6 mm image reconstruction increment. With pitch 1.5, the scan time for a 100-mm scan range is approximately 33 s, and the effective patient dose is approximately 8 mSv. A virtually "frozen" three-dimensional (3D) volume image can be reconstructed in the diastolic phase with a voxel size of about 0.6x0.6x1.0 mm based on a contrast enhanced scan with 1 mm slice collimation and reconstruction with submillimeter image increment. Data from the CTA is transferred to a computer workstation for postprocessing (3D Virtuoso). The method of choice for display is volume rendering (VR) and not surface rendering as used by most investigators for EBCTA. In surface rendering, much of the volumetric data is lost. VR uses the information from all of the voxels in a stack of images in order to create a space-filling picture, meaning data are not lost during the rendering process (Fig. 2). The temporal and spatial resolution of cardiac multi-slice image data even allows for virtual angioscopy of the coronary arteries (Fig. 3).

Non-invasive MSCTA showed a high diagnostic accuracy in the detection and quantification of coronary lesions. The results of MSCT coronary angiography obtained so far from different centers are very encouraging. CTA of the coronary

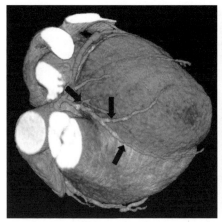 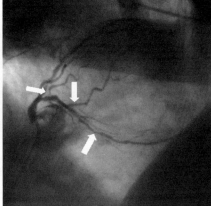

Fig. 2. MSCT angiography of the left anterior descending coronary artery (LAD): detection of a high-grade stenosis in the LAD (*arrow*) and two stenoses at the origins of the diagonal branches (*arrows*). These findings were confirmed with conventional invasive angiography

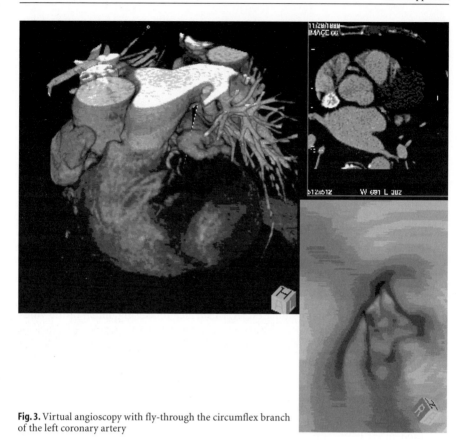

Fig. 3. Virtual angioscopy with fly-through the circumflex branch of the left coronary artery

arteries in 50 patients yielded a sensitivity of 88%, a specificity of 93%, a positive predictive value of 0.91, and a negative predictive value of 0.90 for detection of hemodynamically significant stenoses in the major segments of the coronary arteries [10]. The results revealed a high diagnostic accuracy of MSCT in the detection and quantification of coronary lesions since not only severe but also intermediate and mild lesions could be visualized. The superior spatial resolution allowed depiction of the lumen even in heavily calcified vessels and in vessels with coronary stents. MSCTA yielded excellent results for detection of restenosis after percutaneous coronary angioplasty and for assessment of bypass graft patency [8].

One of the most important findings, however, of the ongoing studies is that MSCTA allowed detection and assessment of noncalcified lipid-rich plaques (Fig. 4). To confirm these findings and to investigate non-invasive detection of coronary plaques and plaque composition using MSCT, intracoronary ultrasound (ICUS) was used as a gold standard. MSCT and ICUS yielded identical results with regard to plaque composition and quantification of lesions [9]. Thus, this new technology holds promise to allow for the non-invasive detection of

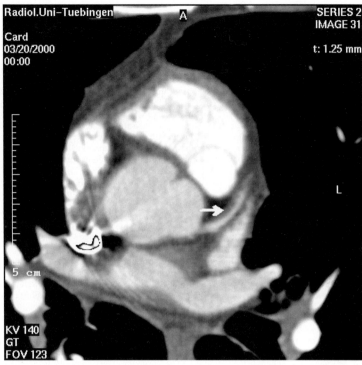

Fig. 4. Noncalcified soft lipid-rich plaque in the left anterior descending coronary artery (LAD; *arrow*). The plaque was confirmed using intracoronary ultrasound

rupture-prone soft coronary lesions and may have the option to lead to early onset of therapy.

Functional Imaging

With ECG-gated multi-slice spiral scanning, 2D or 3D images can be reconstructed in incrementally shifted heart phases with a temporal resolution of up to 125 ms. With multi-planar reformation, the heart can be displayed in any desired plan, such as the short and long axis. This allows functional analysis in a one-stop shopping approach for every patient undergoing CTA of the coronary arteries. From the same spiral data, even a 4D reconstruction of the beating 3D heart that covers a complete heart cycle is feasible [14].

In conclusion, the emergence of superfast MSCT will have a significant impact on cardiac imaging. This new method has the potential to rule out CAD. Now, cardiac calcium scoring, CTA of the coronary arteries, and functional analysis are no longer limited to a dedicated scanner only available at a few major medical centers. Imaging can be performed in a one-stop shopping approach on a standard body CT scanner installed in even minor hospitals. It's obvious that this will have significant impact on the future role of radiologists in cardiac imaging.

References

1. Achenbach S, Moshage W, Ropers D, Nossen J, Daniel WG (1998) Value of electron-beam computed tomography for the noninvasive detection of high-grade coronary-artery stenoses and occlusions. N Engl J Med 339:1964–1971
2. Becker CR, Knez A, Ohnesorge B, Flohr T, Schoepf UJ, Reiser M (1999) Detection and quantification of coronary artery calcifications with prospectively ECG triggered multi-row conventional CT and electron beam computed tomography: comparison of different methods for quantification of coronary artery calcifications. Radiology 213 (P):351
3. Bielak LF, Kaufmann RB, Moll PP, McCollough CH, Schwartz RS, Sheedy PF (1994) Small lesions in the heart identified at electron beam CT: calcification or noise? Radiology 192:631–636
4. Detrano R, Hsiai T, Wang S (1996) Prognostic value of coronary calcification and angiographic stenoses in patients undergoing coronary angiography (abstract). J Am Coll Cardiol 27:285–290
5. Devries S, Wolfkiel CJ, Shah V, Chomka E, Rich S (1995) Reproducibility of the measurement of coronary calcium with ultrafast CT. Am J Cardiol 75:973–975
6. Hernigou A, Challande P, Boudeville JC, Sene V, Grataloup C, Plainfosse MC (1996) Reproducibility of coronary calcification detection with electron-beam computed tomography. Eur Radiol 6:210–216
7. Klingenbeck-Regn K, Schaller S, Flohr T, Ohnesorge B, Kopp AF, Baum U (1999) Subsecond multislice computed tomography: basics and applications. Eur J Radiol 31:110–124
8. Kopp AF. Cardiac Applications of Multidetector-Row CT (1999) 1st International symposium on multidetector-row CT, June 27–28, San Francisco, California (hearing)
9. Kopp AF, Ohnesorge B, Flohr T (1999) High temporal resolution ECG-gated multi-slice spiral CT: a new method for 3D and 4D cardiac imaging (abstract). CVIR 22[suppl]:184
10. Kopp AF, Ohnesorge B, Flohr T, Schroeder S, Claussen CD (1999) Multidetector-row CT for the noninvasive detection of high-grade coronary artery stenoses and occlusions: first results. Radiology 213 (P):435
11. Kopp AF, Ohnesorge B, Flohr T, Georg C, Schröder S, Küttner A, Martensen J, Claussen CD (2000) Multidetektor CT des Herzens: Erste klinische Anwendung einer retrospektiv EKG-gesteuerten Spirale mit optimierter zeitlicher und örtlicher Auflösung zur Darstellung der Herzkranzgefäße. Fortschr.Röntgenstr 172:1–7
12. Moshage WE, Achenbach S, Seese B (1995) Coronary artery stenoses: three-dimensional imaging with electrocardiographically triggered, contrast agent-enhanced, electron-beam CT. Radiology 196:707–714
13. Ohnesorge B, Flohr T, Becker CR, Kopp AF, Knez A (1999) Comparison of EBCT and ECG-gated multislice spiral CT: a study of 3D Ca-scoring with phantom and patient data. Radiology 213:402
14. Ohnesorge B, Flohr T, Becker C, Kopp AF, Schoepf UJ, Baum U, Knez A, Klingenbeck-Regn K, Reiser MF (2000) Cardiac imaging with ECG-gated multi-slice spiral CT – initial experience. Radiology (in press)
15. Shields JP, Mielke-CH J, Rockwood TH, Short RA, Viren FK (1995) Reliability of electron beam computed tomography to detect coronary artery calcification. Am J Card Imaging 9:62–66
16. Thomas PJ, McCollough CH, Ritman EL (1995) An electron-beam CT approach for transvenous coronary arteriography. J Comput Assist Tomogr 19:383–389

Real Time Visualization of Volume Data: Applications in Computed Tomography Angiography

Elliot K. Fishman

The development of 1-s rotation spiral computed tomography (CT), soon followed by subsecond spiral CT (0.75 s) and, more recently, multislice CT (MSCT), represent far more than the ability to acquire more individual scans in a shorter period of time or the ability to complete a scan of a patient in a single breath hold [1, 2]. Rather, the development of these scanners provides, for the first time, true volume data sets which represent the potential for an entirely new paradigm in medical imaging. That is, the ability to scan a chest or abdomen with narrow collimation, in a single breath hold, optimized for contrast enhancement provides an entirely new possibility of our ability to image the patient. This new paradigm is not simply that the use of film is not ideal and that computer-based viewing (PACS network) with a trackball is needed. Rather, it emphasizes that scrolling through a data set with a trackball is also unsatisfactory as the image data set grows from 60 to 100 to 200 to 500 to 1000 images per patient study. Even if a trackball became easier to use and the PACS system more user friendly, a truth would soon emerge. That is that the information seen on axial CT alone is in fact very limited for some applications and totally unsatisfactory for many other applications. While axial images are fine to detect a tumor in the liver, the axial mode might not be ideal in defining the relationship of the tumor to the portal vein, or whether the tumor is resectable for potential cure. Axial images surely are limited for analyzing vascular images, such as a CT angiogram of the aorta, celiac axis, or carotid artery. This limitation is obvious to the radiologist but even more obvious to the referring physician, such as a vascular surgeon, an oncologic surgeon, or a trauma surgeon.

The limitation of an axial display alone is obvious from the magnetic resonance (MR) paradigm, where one of the key added values of MR (especially when comparing MR and CT) always listed is the ability to present the acquired data in any plane, including direct coronal and sagittal imaging. While CT could in fact present axial images reconstructed into the coronal, sagittal, or oblique mode, the reconstructions were limited in quality, especially when the source data was in the 3–4 mm collimation per slice. With the introduction of subsecond spiral CT and most recently MSCT, the potential quality of the data available for coronal and sagittal viewing is better than ever, especially if 1–1.25 mm slice width is used and data reconstructions are at 1-mm intervals. Yet, this still does not take advantage of the full potential of MSCT. To take full advantage of the possibilities of MSCT, the process of review and analysis of CT data must be rethought. When this is done, it becomes clear that the display can no longer be an axial image-based display but must be a true volume display. Only by reviewing data in a true volume will the full potential of CT scanning be realized. Let us then analyze this concept a bit closer.

MSCT scanning allows the user to select the width of the collimators (4 x 1 mm, 4 x 2.5 mm, and 4 x 5 mm), which determine the possible slide widths that can be chosen following scan acquisition. For example, with the four 1-mm collimators, we can create slice thickness of 1, 1.25, 1.5,2, 5, and 10 mm to name a few of the possibilities. Similarly, with the four 2.5-mm collimators we can create slices with a width of 3, 4, 5, or 10 mm to name a few options [3, 4]. When the need for detailed imaging arises, as in cases of CT angiography (CTA), we routinely will use the 4 x 1 mm collimators and reconstruct 1.25-mm thick sections at 1-mm intervals. This provides us not so much a series of slices but a volume of information whether the focus of the volume be the thoracic or abdominal aorta, the celiac axis, or the renal arteries. This volume of information will have a limited value if only reviewed in axial mode and therefore must be reviewed as a volume. This is where real time volume visualization on systems, such as the 3DVirtuoso (Siemens Medical Systems, Erlangen, Germany) creates an entirely new imaging environment.

The 3DVirtuoso, with its real time rendering capability, is the first three-dimensional (3D) workstation designed to focus on the 3D display of volume data sets. The specifics of the 3DVirtuoso are beyond the substance of this chapter, but several technical features need to be reviewed. The system host is a SGI O2 computer custom designed to provide sufficient memory and storage capabilities. In order to handle the large data sets currently being generated by scanners, such as the VolumeZoom (Siemens Medical Systems), an upgrade to the 3DVirtuoso with the Mitsubishi (Boston, Mass.) Volume Pro board and a new operating interface for the 3D interaction is available, which speeds up the rendering by a factor of 15–20 times. This means that data sets of 200–300 images can now be analyzed in real time without the slowing effect seen with large volume data sets. To be more specific, the volume of data is loaded into the memory of the computer, and the user can then decide how that volume is reviewed. Using the technique referred to at volume rendering, a true 3D display accurate to each pixel in the data set can be generated. Depending on the clinical question, a volumetric 3D image can be generated in real time, focusing in on either the soft tissues, bone, or vascular structures to name but a few of the possibilities [5, 6, 7]. The information is viewed in real time by the user and a set of "cut planes" is used to optimize the display of the area in question (i.e., the kidneys and renal arteries in a volume data set of the entire abdomen). Real time editing tools also include a region of interest editing tool, which can quickly remove structures, such as the spine or ribs. The use of real time editing is an important tool for 3D visualization, especially of vascular structures. The need for the editing is especially important in those cases where maximum intensity projection (MIP) images are used.

The use of real time display and editing is a concept that is often looked at as alien and is commonly misunderstood by radiologists. When we discuss real time, we mean that the user can display and select any portion of the scan volume interactively. Any plane or perspective that the user finds helpful can be generated not just select planes, which was the concept with coronal- and sagittal-based imaging typically seen on earlier scanners and/or workstations. When we discuss real time we truly mean that the users interaction with the volume occurs instantaneously and is not delayed by system design or computer under performance. The importance of the real time nature of the system is a core feature as to its usability and acceptance by the radiologic community. We do not feel that a non-real time display will succeed in today's environment. In our paradigm shift, we believe that the radiologist will be the primary user of the real time data and it will become the primary mode of interpretation and consultation. The use of radiologic technologists to do the 3D imaging has been shown to be successful in some institutions, but that is because of the length of time it takes to perform a study on many of the available workstations. With real time rendering, optimal use of the radiologists time is achieved [8]. Another important feature of the real time interactive display is the use of stereo vision to look at images. Anyone who has ever been to Disneyland or Universal Studios knows the impact of quality stereo displays. We currently use a system (CrystalEyes by Stereographics Inc., Mountain View, Calif.) that allows for the real time display of stereo images. Stereo display is especially valuable in complex vascular anatomy and in creating vascular mapping. The value of stereo cannot be underestimated and its one limitation is that the stereo images cannot be captured on print or video for the referring doctor. Viewing is only possible on the workstation.

The use of volume visualization has numerous vascular applications, but a separation of them into categories may make an overview a bit more focused. At John Hopkins Hospital we are currently getting over 50 requests per week for a wide range of vascular applications for 3D CTA. In most of these cases, a CT angiogram is being ordered in the place of other more invasive tests (especially classic catheter based angiography), which provides a cost savings to the enterprise. The significant cost savings (CTA being one-third the cost) of a CT angiogram compared with a classic angiogram have been previously addressed by Rubin et al. [9]. Three major areas of CTA include organ transplant evaluation, oncologic tumor staging, and aneurysm detection/evaluation. Let us look briefly at several examples [10, 11, 12, 13, 14, 15]. It is important to recognize that in each of these cases, the information gained from the 3D CTA maps is far more than the information obtained just by reviewing a set of axial images, whether on film or a workstation. This can be summarized also by saying that the sum is greater than the individual parts.

In our practice, we evaluate all patients who are scheduled to be a living renal donor with CTA. In these cases, the dual phase (arterial and venous phases) CT angiogram provides all of the needed information for the laprascopic harvesting of the kidney. This includes the status of the kidney, the location and number of renal arteries, the location and number of renal veins and the adrenal vein, gonadal veins, and the appearance of the ureter (Fig. 1). Similarly, patients who are potential liver transplant recipients are evaluated with 3D CTA of dual phase CT data acquisitions. This provides information on the status of the liver, the ability to detect or exclude a hepatoma, definition of the hepatic artery and its branches, and the status of the portal vein and the presence of any varices.

Oncologic CT angiograms, with volume rendering provide a comprehensive study that can detect the presence of disease, define the extent of disease, inclu-

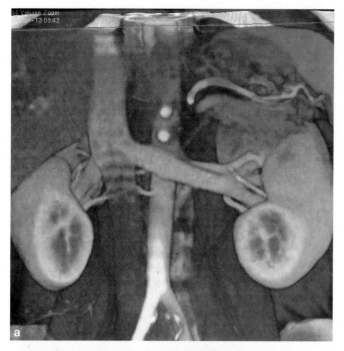

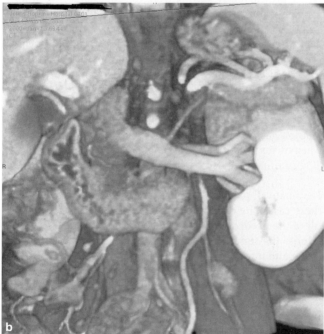

Fig. 1a, b. Three-dimensional reconstructions of a potential renal transplant donor demonstrate normal venous anatomy with a single left renal artery. The left adrenal vein and left gonadal vein are clearly defined

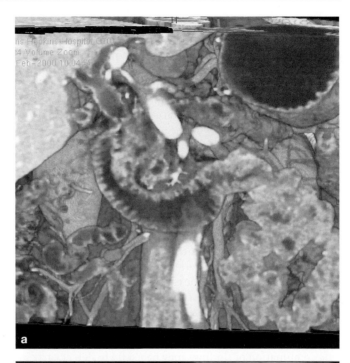

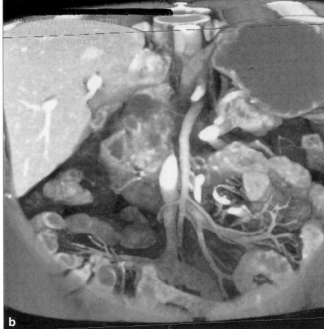

Fig. 2a, b. Three-dimensional reconstructions demonstrate a mass in the pancreatic head consistent with an adenocarcinoma with early duodenal invasion. The superior mesenteric artery (SMA) was patent and the patient was felt to be resectable

ding vessel invasion, and provide vascular maps for surgery. Applications include dual phase CT angiograms for the evaluation of pancreatic tumors, where the 3D map provides detail as to vessel encasement or occlusion that may not be recognized on axial images alone (Fig. 2). The use of the CT angiogram with volume imaging is especially useful in complex cases where it is impossible to distinguish between vessel invasion and simple mass effect by tumor. Similarly, 3D CTA with volume display is used for evaluation of suspected renal masses. In these cases, multi-phase volume acquisitions can define the presence of tumor, its extent, including vascular involvement, and tumor spread. The 3D maps are used for selecting patients for partial nephrectomy.

Classic vascular applications, such as excluding a thoracic and/or abdominal aneurysm or dissection, are becoming mainstream CTA applications (Fig. 3). In these patients, CT provides a rapid study to include or exclude the presence of disease. In addition to defining the extent of an aneurysm or dissection, the data generated using CT is used to design the custom endovascular stents. CTA with volume display is also used to monitor the success of endovascular graft placement and to detect complications with graft leakage.

Other vascular applications where the display of a 3D vascular volume is critical, is the use of 3D CTA for the evaluation of intestinal ischemia. Although this application should be considered more like a works in progress, it is showing great potential. In this application, CTA can not only create vascular maps for analysis but also allow for the concurrent study of bowel enhancement (Fig. 4). The combination of findings may be useful to detect early intestinal ischemia.

There are obviously other vascular applications for CTA, where 3D-volume display is needed. These include the evaluation of suspected pulmonary embolism, coronary artery angiography, and evaluation of peripheral vascular disease. The success of some of these applications will be judged in the near future as the users get more experience.

Despite these obvious paradigm shifts and their clear-cut advantages, the rate of change may not be as fast as one might suspect or hope for. This can be explained by a number of factors, including the fact that these changes will require changes in the workflow pattern; whether it is radiologists' or other professionals' change in workflow, it will not be easy to execute. Whether the reasons for resistance are financial, lack of vision, or simple resistance (who moved my cheese), it will take time and effort to bring these changes about. We are, however, confident that when radiologists look at the advantages of this new imaging paradigm of using volume visualization of the CT data sets, the change will come. The rate of change will obviously be faster if workstation design and performance improve or if radiologists begin to understand how reviewing studies in a volume will improve both their performance and patient outcome. Specific studies will need to be designed to try and measure the impact of change and undoubtedly will be done. Until then, we believe that the excitement will continue with every new advance in scanner design and technology and advances in 3D hardware and software providing impetus for pushing the envelope in medical imaging.

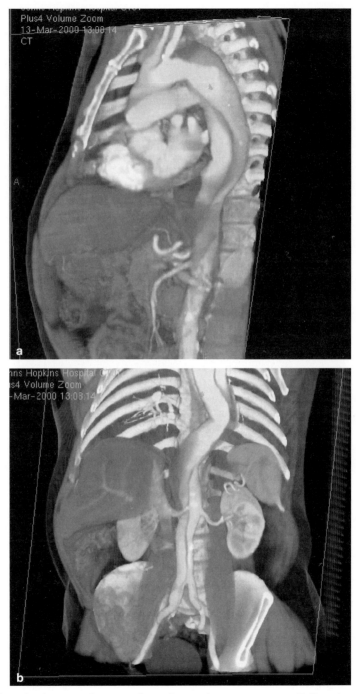

Fig. 3a, b. Three-dimensional computed tomography angiogram demonstrates a type B dissection extending down through abdominal aorta and into the right common iliac artery

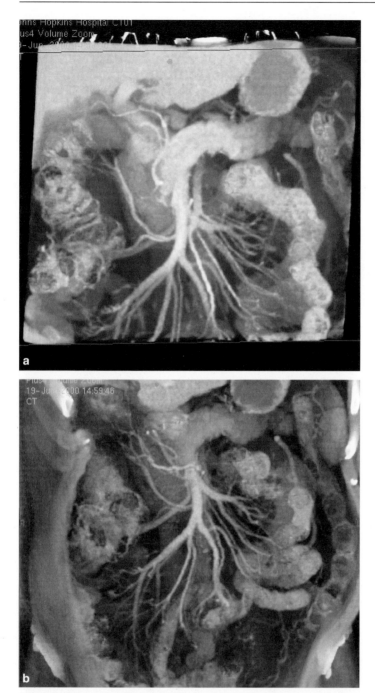

Fig. 4a, b. Three-dimensional computed tomography angiogram of the mesenteric vessels demonstrate several areas of stenosis in the distal branches of the superior mesenteric artery (SMA). Note, however, normal bowel enhancement

References

1. Hu H, He HD, et al. (2000) Four multidetector-row helical CT: image quality and volume coverage speed. Radiology 215:55–62
2. Horton KM, Fishman EK (2000) 3D CT angiography of the celiac and superior mesenteric arteries with multidetector CT data sets: preliminary observations. Abdom Imaging 25:523–525
3. Johnson PT, Fishman EK, et al. (1998) Interactive three-dimensional volume rendering of spiral CT data: current applications in the thorax. Radiographics 18:165–187
4. Kuszyk BS, Fishman EK (1998) Technical aspects of CT angiography. Semin Ultrasound CT MR 19:383–393
5. Calhoun PS, Kuszyk BS, et al. (1999) Three-dimensional volume rendering of spiral CT data: theory and method. Radiographics 19:745–764
6. Kawamoto S, Johnson PT, et al. (1998) Three-dimensional CT angiography of the thorax: clinical applications. Semin Ultrasound CT MR 19:425–438
7. Smith PA, Fishman EK (1998) Three-dimensional CT angiography: renal applications. Semin Ultrasound CT MR 19:413–424
8. Smith PA, Klein AS, et al. (1998) Dual-phase spiral CT angiography with volumetric 3D rendering for preoperative liver transplant evaluation: preliminary observations. J Comput Assist Tomogr 22:868–874
9. Rubin GD, et al. (2000) Cost identification of abdominal aortic aneurysm imaging by using time and motion analysis. Radiology 215:63–70
10. Rubin GD, Shiau MC, et al. (1999) Computed tomographic angiography: historical perspective and new state-of-the-art using multidetector-row helical computed tomography. J Comput Tomogr 23[suppl 1]:83–90
11. Coll DM, Uzzo RG, et al. (1999) 3-dimensional volume rendered computerized tomography for preoperative evaluation and intraoperative treatment of patients undergoing nephron-sparing surgery. J Urol 161:1097–1002
12. Remy-Jardin M, Remy J (1999) Spiral CT angiography of the pulmonary circulation. Radiology 212:615–636
13. Smith PA, Marshall FF, et al. (1999) Planning nephron-sparing renal surgery using 3D helical CT angiography. J Comput Assist Tomogr 23:649–654
14. Johnson PT, Halpern EJ, et al. (1999) Renal artery stenosis: CT angiography–comparison of real-time volume-rendering and maximum intensity projection algorithms. Radiology 211:337–343
15. Wu CM, Urban BA, et al. (1999) Spiral CT of the thoracic aorta with 3-D volume rendering: A pictorial review of current applications. Cardiovasc Intervent Radiol 22:159–167

Fast High-Resolution Computed Tomography Angiography of Peripheral Vessels

Carlo Catalano, Andrea Grossi, Alessandro Napoli, Francesco Fraioli

Introduction

Obstructive arterial disease of the lower extremities is an extremely common disease in western countries that requires an accurate diagnosis for a correct treatment planning. The examination of choice for the assessment of patients with obstructive arterial disease is X-ray angiography, which allows for the correct demonstration of arterial anatomy. Nevertheless, its invasiveness has led to the development of non-invasive examinations. In many arterial districts, X-ray angiography has been progressively substituted by non-invasive examinations, among which are magnetic resonance angiography (MRA) and computed tomography angiography (CTA). In the assessment of the peripheral arterial district, due to the length of the volume to be examined, CTA could not be proposed because of technical limitations. On the contrary, contrast-enhanced MRA (c.e.) provides excellent results in a fairly short acquisition time and has increasingly substituted X-ray angiography in several centers.

The recent development of multislice CT (MSCT) has totally changed and improved the technique of CTA. In fact, the possibility of scanning large volumes allows routine examinations of arterial districts which could not previously be examined using single slice spiral CTA. Furthermore, in multislice spiral CTA, some of the limitations of single slice spiral CTA, such as the use of large doses of iodinated contrast agent and the high X-ray dose to the patient, are being reduced due to the speed of acquisition (smaller doses of contrast agent) and technical improvements (reduction of X-ray dose to the patient).

Optimization of the Technique

Patient Positioning

Patients can be indifferently positioned with their feet or head first. Nevertheless, a wider volume can be examined positioning the patient supine with feet first. In fact, the movement of the table does not allow, when the patient is positioned with the head first, one to reach the distal tract of the thigh vessels and the ankles with the examination volume, even if the patient is not particularly tall. On the contrary, if the patient is positioned with feet first, it is possible to widen the examination volume down to the ankles and, if necessary, down the pedal circu-

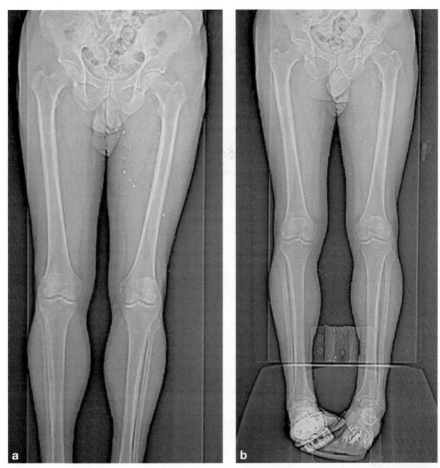

Fig. 1a, b. A greater volume can be acquired positioning the patient with the feet first (**b**), compared with the head first (a). The introversion of the feet allows the separation of the tibia from the fibula

lation (Fig. 1). It is furthermore important, exactly like it is advisable in conventional arteriography, to tie the patient's feet in introversion in order to separate the tibia from the fibula (Fig. 1) and, as a consequence, the trifurcation vessels, which have a course parallel to the bony structures. The separation of vessels from bony structures is essential to simplify the three-dimensional (3D) reconstructions following the acquisition. In order to avoid even minimal motion artifacts during the acquisition, it is advisable to tie the patient's feet.

Scanning Protocol

After a 1024-mm initial topogram, the acquisition volume is positioned in such a way to comprise all arterial structures from the suprarenal abdominal aorta down

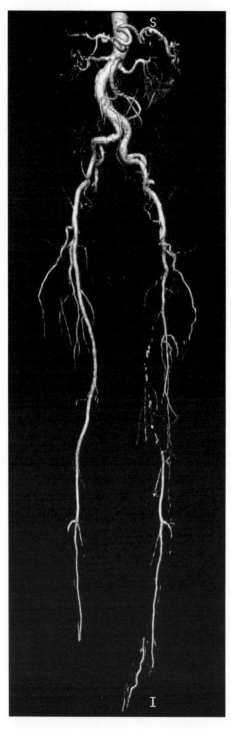

Fig. 2. The 120-cm volume of acquisition allows the coverage of arterial segments from the renal arteries down to the ankles

to the ankles, reaching if possible, also the feet (Fig. 2). The largest possible volume is 120 cm at the moment, which is sufficient in most of the cases. The actual limitation, in terms of examination volume, is related to the motion of the table, which can be exploited to the maximum, as previously said, if the patient is positioned with feet first. The protocol we use consists of a 4 x 2.5-mm collimation with a slice thickness of reconstructed images of 3 mm. The reconstruction interval is 3 mm. It derives that in order to cover 120 cm, the scanning time is 40 s, during which approximately 400 images are produced. If necessary, the acquired volume can then be reconstructed at different slice thicknesses and/or different reconstruction intervals. In particular, in order to obtain a greater detail, especially at the level of the origin of the renal arteries and of the distal trifurcation vessels, images are reconstructed with a slice interval of 1 mm, which means an overlap of 2 mm.

Intravenous Administration of the Contrast Agent

In order to obtain a good CTA examination of the peripheral arteries, a correct intravenous administration of the iodinated contrast agent is crucial. A 17–18 gauge IV cannula must be inserted in an antecubital vein; its patency is verified with a flush of saline solution. Different types of iodinated contrast agents can be utilized in CTA. In our experience, the best results are obtained with a high iodine concentration contrast agent (400 mgI/ml). In fact, the comparison of contrast agents with a lower concentration of iodine (300 mgI/ml and 350 mgI/ml), has shown an increase of arterial enhancement directly proportional to the concentration of iodine in the contrast agent, maintaining the same overall amount of iodine injected (40 g of I per examination; see chapter on contrast agents).

Regarding the flow velocity, the best results are obtained with a flow rate of 4 ml/s, with a uniphasic injection. At the beginning of our experience on the multi-slice CT, no technique for calculation of the patient delay time (test bolus or bolus chasing) was available. Therefore, in order to utilize a fixed delay time of 25–28 s in all patients, it was decided empirically and standardized based on previous experiences with single slice spiral CT and MRA. In less than 5% of the more than 120 patients examined until now with this method, the arterial opacification was inadequate. In the case of young patients, the delay time can be reduced by a few seconds. In general, in patients with obstructive arterial disease and claudicatio, a fixed delay time can be satisfactorily utilized. Nevertheless, if the clinical suspicion is an aneurysmal disease (i.e., popliteal artery aneurysm), the delay time may be prolonged at the level of the dilatation and it can be considered to use a longer delay time or to calculate the delay time by means of a test bolus if available. There has been no venous enhancement overlying arterial segments that impaired the image quality in any of the cases.

3D Reconstructions

A large amount of data is routinely produced with a MSCT when a peripheral vascular study is performed. Generally, 400–600 images are obtained in each examination and if further reconstructions are performed, for instance at the level of the renal arteries or the trifurcation vessels, the number can become even greater. In consideration of the huge amount of data available, a simple and reliable 3D reconstruction method should be used. In the peripheral district, arterial segments run close to bony structures, particularly at the level of the calves, and therefore they should be eliminated to obtain a better 3D display. This can be obtained by performing a vascular segmentation, which can become time consuming but then allows images to be visualized with different reconstruction algorithms, such as MIP (maximum intensity projection), SSD (surface shaded display) and VR (volume rendering). Otherwise, in order to avoid the segmentation process and reduce the reconstruction time, it is possible to perform reconstructions with VR, which provides a perspective view, allowing the differentiation of bony structures from vascular structures. In our institution, the VR technique is routinely utilized without any vascular segmentation. By doing so, the process requires approximately 10 min on a dedicated workstation with experienced personnel. In all cases, anterior, posterior, lateral, and oblique views are obtained.

Image Analysis

In the evaluation of a run-off study, it is always necessary together with the visualization of 3D reconstructions to rapidly scroll all of the transverse images to obtain more accurate information on the degree of stenosis, morphology of the plaque, and presence of aneurysmal disease. Scrolling of the images takes only a very short time with the possibility to stop and take a better look at regions of interest.

Clinical Results

Several studies have shown the high accuracy of single slice spiral CTA in the assessment of vascular pathologies in several districts; nevertheless, the technique could not be applied in the evaluation of the peripheral circulation due to the size of the volume to be examined. MSCT has made these studies possible and, although there are no studies yet published on the topic, the results appear to be encouraging. In fact, the technique simply exploits the passage of the contrast agent through the arterial vessels. Our early results show an excellent correlation with X-ray angiography, which is greater at the level of the aorto-iliac tract (Fig. 3) and slightly and increasingly lower at the level of the thigh (Fig. 4) and calf (Fig. 5), where the caliber of the arteries is significant reduced. The largest part of diagnostic errors happened to be in the early phase of the experience either because of overestimation or underestimation. In particular, the latter is caused by the presence of diffuse calcifications and may be avoided by an attentive analysis, especially utilizing different types of reconstruction algorithms and, if necessary, going back to transverse images. In such a way, it is possible to detect the residual patent lumen and better quantify the degree of stenosis.

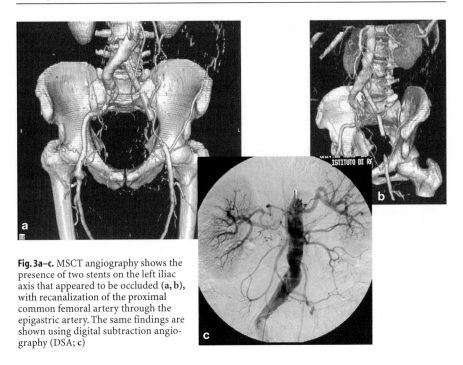

Fig. 3a–c. MSCT angiography shows the presence of two stents on the left iliac axis that appeared to be occluded (**a, b**), with recanalization of the proximal common femoral artery through the epigastric artery. The same findings are shown using digital subtraction angiography (DSA; **c**)

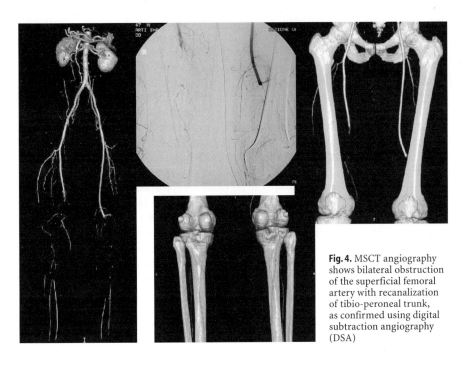

Fig. 4. MSCT angiography shows bilateral obstruction of the superficial femoral artery with recanalization of tibio-peroneal trunk, as confirmed using digital subtraction angiography (DSA)

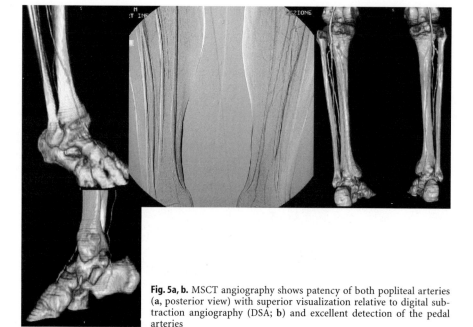

Fig. 5a, b. MSCT angiography shows patency of both popliteal arteries (**a**, posterior view) with superior visualization relative to digital subtraction angiography (DSA; **b**) and excellent detection of the pedal arteries

CTA presents several advantages over X-ray angiography. First, it is totally noninvasive. Although X-ray angiography has become a safe procedure, it still requires an arterial approach, which requires immobilization of the patient for at least a few hours and may carry some complications. Furthermore, its costs are quite high. Second, its costs are limited; the examination can be easily standardized and the overall examination time is very short (5 min, comprising patient positioning and insertion of an IV cannula). The CT examination is very well accepted by all patients and the exam did not have to be interrupted for any reason in any of the cases. Another advantage is the superior visualization of collaterals in the presence of obstructions and severe stenoses and distal vessels. Routinely, the trifurcation vessels are opacified and in most cases pedal vessels are also shown. At the level of the foot, there might be some technical problems in 3D reconstructions due to the very close course of vessels with bones. Some automatic reconstruction techniques may be particularly useful for the 3D display of distal vessels. Furthermore, in CTA, differences in circulation time between the two lower limbs are generally not significant like they are in X-ray angiography. In none of the cases examined until now in our institution has there been an inadequate opacification of arterial segments. This is in contrast with X-ray angiography. The main reason is that the scanning time is relatively prolonged, allowing visualization also of distal vessels (trifurcation vessels are generally examined 1 min from initiation of the IV contrast agent administration) but also the transverse plane allows superior resolution.

If necessary, the scanning protocol can be modified with reduction of the slice collimation and increase of the spatial resolution; routinely it appears to us that a

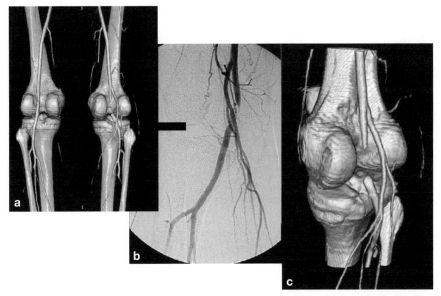

Fig. 6a–c. Popliteal entrapment: MSCT angiography on a posterior view (**a, b**) shows compression of the left popliteal artery during stress, as confirmed using digital subtraction angiography (DSA; **c**, anterior view)

2.5 collimation is sufficient for display of peripheral arteriopathies. Nevertheless, in some cases, in which a superior detail is needed or limited segments have to be examined, a high-resolution protocol can be utilized. This is the case with arterial extrinsic compressions (popliteal entrapment or others; Fig. 6) or diabetic arteriopathies (necessity to examine pedal vessels for potential distal bypasses).

The other non-invasive technique that provides a direct visualization of arterial districts is c.e. MRA, which also provides excellent results, similar to those of multislice CTA. Nevertheless peripheral MRA is quite complicated to perform and it requires, in order to obtain a detailed examination, dedicated hardware and software: moving beds and dedicated coils are available only in a small percentage of equipment. Even if sophisticated systems are utilized, there are still some limitations in terms of spatial resolution, particularly in distal vessels. The cost of the MRA examination is significantly superior to the CTA, mainly due to the paramagnetic contrast media, which is significantly more expensive than iodinated agents. The examination time in MRA can be prolonged, particularly in those cases in which transverse images (c.e. MRA is acquired in the coronal plane) are also needed (aneurysmal disease).

The main advantages of MRA are the use of non-ionizing radiation and non-nephrotoxic contrast agents. Nevertheless, there has been a significant reduction in X-ray dose to the patient when using multislice CTA compared with previous equipment and further reductions are expected, while iodinated contrast media are quickly becoming safer, with minimal adverse reactions. Both techniques are undoubtedly extremely valid and are already now able to substitute, in most instances, catheter angiography, also in emergency cases (particularly CTA).

In conclusion, multislice CTA, although only very recently developed and introduced in the clinical practice, appears to be a valid and reliable technique for the assessment of peripheral arterial disease. Further improvements are expected for what concerns the acquisition and especially for the 3D reconstruction process.

Suggested Reading

1. Hu H, He HD, Foley WD, Fox SH (2000) Four multidetector-row helical CT: image quality and volume coverage speed. Radiology 215:55–62
2. Rubin GD, Shiau MC, Leung AN, Kee ST, Logan LJ, Sofilos MC (2000) Aorta and iliac arteries: single versus multiple detector-row helical CT angiography. Radiology 215:670–676
3. Fleischmann D, Rubin GD, Bankier AA, Hittmair K (2000) Improved uniformity of aortic enhancement with customized contrast medium injection protocols at CT angiography. Radiology 214: 363–371
4. Rubin GD, Shiau MC, Schmidt AJ, et al. (1999) Computed tomographic angiography: historical perspective and new state-of-the-art using multi detector-row helical computed tomography. J Comput Assist Tomogr 23[suppl 1]:83–90
5. Hu H (1999) Multi-slice helical CT: scan and reconstruction. Med Phys 26:5–18
6. Rubin GD, Walker PJ, Dake MD, et al (1993) 3D spiral CT angiography: an alternative imaging modality for the abdominal aorta and its branches. J Vasc Surg 18:656–666
7. Rubin GD, Napel SA, Ringl H, Brosnan TJ (1996) Assessment of section profile and clinical images in helical CT with pitch values of 0.5–3.0 by using 180° linear extrapolation and segmented reconstruction (abstract). Radiology 201:246
8. Polacin A, Kalender WA, Marchal G (1992) Evaluation of section sensitivity profiles and image noise in spiral CT. Radiology 185:29–35
9. Rubin GD, Napel S (1995) Increased scan pitch for vascular and thoracic spiral CT. Radiology 197:316–317
10. Fishman EK (1997) High-resolution three-dimensional imaging from subsecond helical CT data sets: applications in vascular imaging. AJR Am J Roentgenol 169:441–443
11. Dillon EH, van Leeuwen MS, Fernandez MA, Mali WP (1993) Spiral CT angiography. AJR Am J Roentgenol 160:1273–1278
12. Klingenbeck-Regn K, Schaller S, Flohr T, Ohnesorge B, Kopp AF, Baum U (1999) Subsecond multislice computed tomography: basics and applications. Eur J Radiol 31:110–124
13. McCollough CH, Zink FE (1999) Performance evaluation of a multi-slice CT system. Med Phys 26:2223–2230
14. Tierney S, Fennessy F, Hayes DB (2000) ABC of arterial and vascular disease. Secondary prevention of peripheral vascular disease. BMJ 320:1262–1265
15. Dormandy J, Heeck L, Vig S (1999) Predictors of early disease in the lower limbs. Semin Vasc Surg 12:109–117
16. Dormandy J, Heeck L, Vig S (1999) Peripheral arterial occlusive disease: clinical data for decision making. Introduction. Semin Vasc Surg 12:95
17. Leiner T, Ho KY, Nelemans PJ, de Haan MW, van Engelshoven JM (2000) Three-dimensional contrast-enhanced moving-bed infusion-tracking (MoBI-track) peripheral MR angiography with flexible choice of imaging parameters for each field of view. J Magn Reson Imaging 11:368–377
18. Semba CP, Murphy TP, Bakal CW, Calis KA, Matalon TA (2000) Thrombolytic therapy with use of alteplase (rt-PA) in peripheral arterial occlusive disease: review of the clinical literature. The Advisory Panel. J Vasc Interv Radiol 11:149–161

IV Multislice Computed Tomography Applications in the Chest

Multislice Computed Tomography of the Lung Parenchyma

Mathias Prokop

Introduction

Computed tomography (CT) is still the most important imaging technique for diseases of the lung parenchyma. Spiral CT has taken this technique form a mere cross-sectional modality to a volumetric imaging tool and has markedly improved the detection of small pulmonary nodules, the staging of lung tumors, and the evaluation of the tracheobronchial system. Multi-planar reformations (MPRs) that were able to demonstrate the longitudinal extent of disease and allow for sections that could be individually adapted to pathology became possible. However, these reformations suffered from a limited spatial resolution if the spiral scan had to cover the whole chest. Alternatively, spiral CT provided high-resolution images but at the cost of a substantially reduced scan coverage. High-resolution CT (HRCT) and spiral CT remained reserved for distinctly different indications (apart from some fringe applications). Thus, evaluation of focal and diffuse lung disease in the same patient required two separate scan protocols to be performed after each other.

Multislice CT (MSCT) is a new technology that mends a lot of the residual drawbacks of spiral CT. It provides near isotropic data sets of the whole chest that allow for true multi-planar imaging with nearly identical image quality in any desired imaging plane without compromising the coverage of the scan [1]. It is the first technology that allows for high-resolution coronal or axial sections of the lung parenchyma in situ. It simultaneously provides data for the evaluation of focal lung disease and for high-resolution imaging of diffuse lung disorders. MSCT therefore offers a number of new, exciting opportunities for imaging of the lung parenchyma.

Technique

In MSCT, scanning (data acquisition) is much more separated form data reconstruction than in spiral CT, because MSCT allows for reconstruction of almost any arbitrary section thickness as long as it is larger than the minimum resulting from the chosen scan protocol [1].

Spatial Resolution

Spatial resolution in spiral CT is limited by the speed of the scanner. Within a 30-s breath-holding phase, standard 1-s spiral CT scanners can only perform 30 rotations. Given a scan range of 24 cm, this requires a scanning protocol that uses 8 mm table feed per tube rotation, resulting in an effective section width [full width at half maximum (FWHM)] of 5.9 mm if a section collimation of 5 mm is used. Thin-section scanning with 1-mm collimation and 2 mm table feed is only able to cover a range of 6 cm with 1-s spiral CT scanners. Even with subsecond scanners (0.75 s tube rotation), this scán range can only be increased to some 8 cm. Therefore, scanning with spiral CT is always a compromise between scan length and effective section width.

MSCT using the SOMATOM Volume Zoom can cover a range of 24 cm in some 20 s even though 1-mm sections are employed. The effective section width with this protocol is merely 1.25 mm. With a field of view of 30–40 cm for the chest, the pixel size on axial images is in the 0.6–0.8 mm range. Thus, overlapping reconstruction every 0.6–0.8 mm will yield an isotropic set of three-dimensional (3D) data points. Of course, the spatial resolution still is not fully isotropic because each of these data point samples information from a longer portion (FWHM 1.25 mm) along the z-axis. The thin sections substantially reduce partial volume averaging, improve the display of fine structures, and allow for excellent MPRs even for coronal or sagittal sections.

Using a faster protocol with 4 x 2.5 mm, the effective section width is 3.0 mm, but the scan time scan be substantially decreased to some 8 s for the complete chest. Protocols with even larger collimation play no role for imaging of the chest. In the following section, these two main protocols will be discussed.

High-Resolution Protocol ('Thin Collimation')

High-resolution scan protocols can be recommended as the standard for most high-end indications in the chest. This includes all situations in which multi-planar sections may be required (tumor staging or characterization), imaging of the tracheobronchial system, and examinations in which both, focal and diffuse lung diseases, have to be evaluated.

A high-resolution protocol is based on a 4 x 1-mm collimation ('thin collimation' protocol on the SOMATOM Volume Zoom) and covers the whole chest. For most indications in the chest, the pitch factor is of minor importance. In general, a pitch of 5–8 can be recommended. The advantage of a high pitch is the increased scanning speed (at a pitch of 8, 15-s scan time is required for a range of 24 cm), but this comes at the cost of slightly increased artifacts in the periphery of the scan field [1]. These artifacts result in tiny steps that spiral around the center of the gantry and can best be appreciated at the pleural surface and the rib contours on coronal reformations. As a consequence, a pitch factor of 8 may be best suited for dyspneic patients, while for most other patients, lower pitch factors around 6 can be recommended [2].

High-Speed Protocol ('Fast')

A high-speed scan protocol ('fast' on the SOMATOM Volume Zoom) is based on a 4 x 2.5-mm collimation and provides a very rapid evaluation of the chest with a somewhat reduced spatial resolution. As mentioned previously, the acquisition of the chest (24-cm scan range) takes only about 8 s at a pitch of 6, which makes the technique attractive in patients that cannot hold their breath well. The effective section width is 3 mm, and thus is still markedly better than with spiral CT. MPRs are, therefore, also superior to spiral CT but do not provide the excellent detail seen with the high-resolution protocol.

The high-speed protocol may serve as a standard technique for imaging of the lung parenchyma in a routine situation (e.g., screening for chest metastases, follow-up after therapy). It is especially helpful in critically ill and dyspneic patients since scan time is so short.

Data Reconstruction

Data reconstruction in MSCT is separated from data acquisition more than in spiral CT. The width of the reconstructed sections (effective section width = FWHM of the section sensitivity profile) and the reconstruction interval can be chosen independently from the acquisition parameters as long as the effective section width is equal to or larger than the minimum available with the chosen scanning parameters (1.25 mm with the high-resolution protocol and 3.0 mm with the high-speed protocol) [1].

Standard Axial Images

For almost all indications of MSCT of the lung parenchyma, an effective section width of 5 mm can be recommended for axial images (Fig. 1a), reconstructed in an overlapping fashion every 3 mm. This procedure is possible both with the high-resolution and the high-speed protocol. It has the advantage that the total number of images is around 80, which makes the data set easy to handle with present workstations and even allows for printout of every second image on 20-on-1 format hardcopies (two films).

This approach is a sufficient way of presenting axial images for the vast majority of patients. A moderately high-resolution kernel (e.g., B60) should be employed for image reconstruction, because it poses a compromise between image noise and spatial resolution.

HRCT/Combi Scan

In those cases in which there is the suspicion of a diffuse lung disease, additional 1.25-mm thick high-resolution scans (Fig. 1b) may be reconstructed every 10 mm, very much the same way as in conventional HRCT [2, 3]. This, however, requires that the data set be acquired with 4 x 1-mm collimation. Using this approach, MSCT is able to yield both overlapping axial sections and high-resolution images ('combi scan').

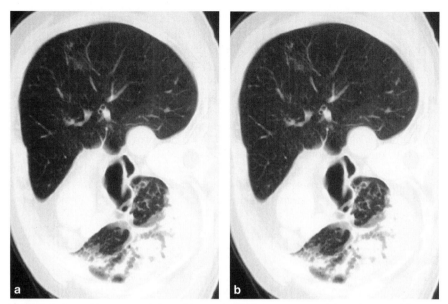

Fig. 1a, b. Patient with poststenotic bronchiectases after sleeve resection of the right upper lobe. A 5-mm section for a data set obtained with a high-resolution protocol (**a**) is compared with a 1.25-mm high-resolution computed tomography (HRCT) section (**b**) from the same data set. Note the improved demonstration of the septal stenosis (*arrow*) and the better definition of the ectatic and thickened bronchial walls and the centrilobular emphysema

Secondary Raw Data Set

Multi-planar imaging with near isotropic resolution requires the use of a high-resolution protocol. In order to obtain an isotropic set of data points, axial sections of 1.25 mm effective section width are reconstructed every 0.6–0.8 mm. For the lung parenchyma, the highest quality multi-planar images are obtained if a moderately high-resolution kernel (B60) is employed for the reconstruction of this set of overlapping axial images. Since this set of images is too large (300–400 images) to be evaluated section by section and often also suffers from too high an image noise (especially in obese patients, due to the small section thickness), it has to be subjected to further processing and can thus be mainly considered as a 'secondary raw data set'.

Multi-Planar Images

Multi-planar images from the secondary raw data set can be reconstructed in any desired imaging plane (including axial sections) [3]. These multi-planar reformats need not be only one pixel thick but can be reconstructed at any desired thickness as long as this section thickness exceeds the pixel size (coronal or sagittal reformations) or the effective section width (axial reformations).

For imaging of the lung parenchyma, coronal and sagittal sections of 1.5 mm width are best suited to demonstrate the interlobar fissures and interstitial

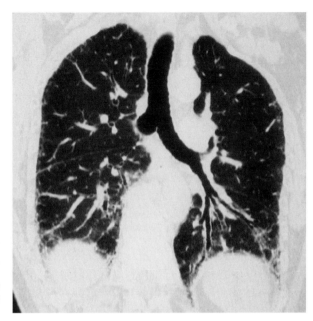

Fig. 2. Coronal 1.5-mm thick high-resolution computed tomography (HRCT) section in a patient with idiopathic pulmonary fibrosis. Note the excellent display of the predominant involvement of the lung periphery and the bases of both lungs

abnormalities (Fig. 2). These high-resolution sections need to be reconstructed only every 3–5 mm, depending on whether a focal or a diffuse abnormality was seen on the axial sections. For optimum results, coronal sections should be slightly tilted anteriorly in order to run parallel to the course of the trachea.

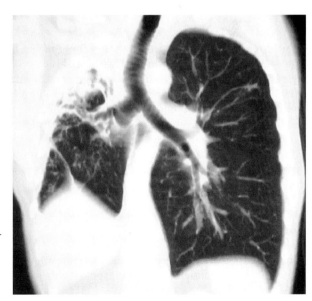

Fig. 3. Slightly tilted 10-mm thick coronal section from the same data set as Fig. 1. Note the excellent demonstration of the central tracheobronchial system and the high-grade stenosis of the remaining middle lobe after sleeve resection of the right upper lobe

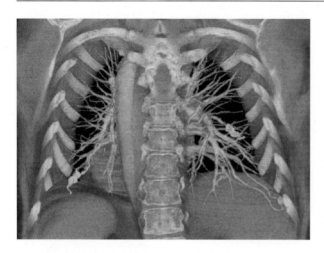

Fig. 4. Volume-rendered data set from a patient with Osler's disease and multiple arteriovenous malformations (AVMs). Some of these AVMs were already embolized with platinum coils. Note the excellent overview over these multiple abnormalities

For imaging of the bronchial system, thicker sections yield a better anatomic overview (5 mm for the peripheral bronchi, 10 mm for the central tracheobronchial system; Fig. 3). Thicker sections are also superior for hilar and mediastinal disease because they reduce image noise. Instead of axial images, coronal sections have been suggested as the primary mode for making the diagnosis. In this case, the whole chest has to be covered. A section thickness of 3–5 mm reconstructed every 3 mm appears most suitable for this imaging task. Interactive cuts may become necessary to optimally display the structure of interest/details of pathologic findings. Again, a section thickness of 1.5–2 mm is best suited for the lung parenchyma.

Volume Rendering

Volume rendering is a 3D visualization technique that is excellent for demonstrating the anatomic relationships of abnormalities, vessels, and bronchi (Fig. 4). However, other than for vessels, it rarely provides additional information over MPRs. On the contrary, it is much more susceptible to image noise and requires sufficiently high patient dose to obtain a good image quality.

With the new version of the 'Virtuoso' workstation, real-time interactive rendering is so fast that it may substitute for other display techniques, including MPRs. In this scenario, however, there remains a problem with adequate documentation of the complete examination unless the whole 3D evaluation procedure is documented on video.

Dose Requirements

For imaging of the lung parenchyma, 60–100 mA (effective mA) at 120 kVp is sufficient in most patients. This corresponds with a mean organ dose in the chest of 8–13 mGy [weighted CT dose index ($CTDI_w$)]. If mediastinal imaging is also required, as is the case in most patients, one may consider reconstructing the data set a second time with a softer filter kernel (B30), either only as thick axial sections or as another secondary raw data set from which thick coronal or sagittal reformations are reconstructed.

Low-Dose CT

Low-dose CT of the lung parenchyma is possible using 10–40 mA (CTDI$_w$ = 1–5 mGy), depending on the size of the patients. Most authors suggest the use of a high-speed protocol (less dose), but high-resolution protocols offer the opportunity to obtain high quality coronal images (if the section thickness of these coronal MPRs is increased to 5 mm or more). Using two separate filter kernels for the lungs (B50) and the mediastinum (B20) allows for sufficient image quality despite the low patient dose (Fig. 5).

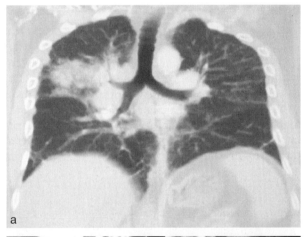

a

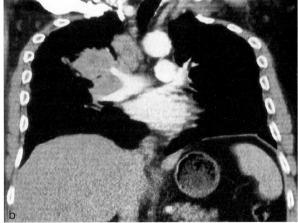

Fig. 5a, b. Low-dose multislice computed tomography (20 mA) in a moderately obese patient with sarcoid disease who developed a bronchogenic carcinoma of the right upper lobe. The 'secondary raw data sets' for the coronal reformations were reconstructed with different filter kernels for the lungs (a) and the soft tissues (b)

b

Patient Preparation and Scanning Direction

For imaging of the lungs, the tracheobronchial system should be free of mucus, because CT often cannot differentiate between a focal collection of mucus and a tumor or polypoid lesion. Thus, the patient should be encouraged to cough immediately prior to the exam. Scanning in a caudocranial direction is useful because it reduces the amount of breathing artifacts if the patient can no longer hold the breath close to the end of the scan.

Clinical Applications

There are a wide variety of diseases whose diagnosis may profit from the use of MSCT. However, since the technique is still new, very little has been published to date.

Anatomy/Localization of Pathology

The demonstration of anatomic detail is excellent with MSCT. In particular, the evaluation of pulmonary fissures becomes much easier, especially if MPRs (coronal and sagittal) are employed. Incomplete fissures are a very frequent finding (Fig. 6) that may have pathologic relevance because disease processes may either be contained in complete fissures or spread across incomplete fissures.

The multi-planar imaging capabilities also improve the localization of pathologic processes: nodules or masses may be better attributed to a pulmonary lobe or segment, and there is better differentiation between pleural and parenchymal disease in difficult cases.

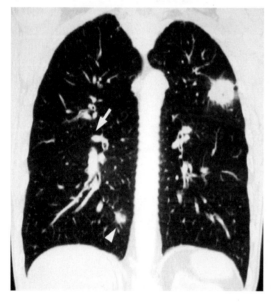

Fig. 6. Coronal reformation of a patient with a bronchogenic carcinoma of the left upper lobe and a secondary nodule (*arrow head*) in the right lower lobe. Note the presence of an incomplete minor fissure (*arrow*)

Lung Nodules

Nodule detection is already excellent with spiral CT, even if thicker sections are used [4]. MSCT may further improve detection rates for small nodules (<5 mm). Such nodules, however, can be found in most patients and in the majority of cases are benign [5]. There is still no consensus on how to handle these findings. MSCT will further increase this problem.

Nodule Characterization

MSCT is not only able to detect more nodules, but may also aid in distinguishing benign from malignant disease. There are known imaging features that suggest malignancy, which were established for thin-section spiral CT scans [6]. MSCT with a high-resolution protocol automatically yields the necessary data to perform such a morphologic analysis (Fig. 6). However, there is still quite an overlap between benign and malignant nodules. Close follow-up (3–6 months) with volumetric analysis of these nodules, as suggested in the lung cancer screening trials [7], may be a way of determining whether to biopsy or resect such a nodule.

Bronchogenic Carcinoma

Staging of bronchogenic carcinoma is based on CT, bronchoscopy, biopsy, and mediastinoscopy. CT is excellent for staging of peripheral bronchial carcinomas but may encounter problems with more extensive or central tumors and with staging of lymph node involvement [8]. Improvements in performance were described for CT with thin collimation and can be expected to be similar or superior if MSCT with a high-resolution protocol is employed.

Spiral CT with thin sections was shown to be advantageous for evaluation of transfissural growth [9]; while the sensitivity for the presence of extension through the major fissure was 57% for thick 10 mm sections, it could be increased to 87% with thin 2 mm sections. Additional MPRs could improve sensitivity to 100%. For the minor fissure, 6 of 51 cases were inconclusive upon axial section but only one remained so upon MPR.

The evaluation of pleural dissemination also profited from thin sections [10]; the sensitivity could be increased from 50% (10 of 20 patients) to 90% with thin 2-mm sections. Accuracy improved from 78% to 93%. Thus, MSCT can be expected to substantially improve the evaluation of more advanced tumor stages. The relationship of a tumor to the pulmonary fissures or transfissural growth is exquisitely demonstrated. The evaluation of invasion of the chest wall or mediastinum can be expected to benefit as well. Due to its excellent spatial resolution along all three imaging planes, CT may even outperform magnetic resonance imaging (MRI) for this imaging task.

Limitations of MSCT result from the pure availability of morphologic criteria. The differentiation between small cell and other lung cancers will always require biopsy. Positron emission tomography (PET) scanning will remain superior when it comes to evaluation of tumor spread to the mediastinum, pleura, and distant sites. MSCT, however, will substantially aid in choosing the right targets for further interventions and will remain the most important tool for surgical planning.

Lymph Node Staging

Shimoyama et al. found that thin section imaging of the hilar lymph nodes improves diagnostic accuracy to 88% if not only the size criterion (usually >10 mm in smallest diameter) but also morphologic criteria are employed [11]. Of the locations with normal lymph nodes, 95% had a straight or concave pleural interface with the lungs, while 95% of locations with malignant lymph nodes had a convex interface. This led to an improvement in sensitivity from 50% for the size criterion to 87%, while specificity only slightly changed from 80% to 83%.

Even for the evaluation of hilar and mediastinal lymph nodes, a substantial improvement of the dismal performance of standard CT can be expected. Here, the main advantage will result from additional morphologic criteria, such as the bulging of the pleural line or the ratio between the minimum and maximum diameter of a lymph node. This criterion has only now become available because MSCT allows for measurement of lymph node size in all three spatial planes. However, secure differentiation between hyperplastic nodules and lymph node metastases will never be perfect when using morphologic criteria only.

Bronchial Carcinoma Screening/Low-Dose MSCT

There is a growing interest in lung cancer screening using CT in a highly selected population of high-risk smokers. Low-dose spiral CT of the lung parenchyma is performed to detect lung nodules [12]. If a nodule is seen, an additional high-resolution scan has to be performed for characterization and follow-up [6].

Low-dose MSCT using a high-resolution protocol offers the advantage that nodules not only can be detected but also can be further evaluated without having to scan the patient again. Using a smoothing filter kernel for the mediastinum (as described above), even the mediastinal lymph nodes can often be evaluated from the same scan (Fig. 5).

Pulmonary Vessels

Peripheral pulmonary vessels can be evaluated without contrast material and are best appreciated on thin-slab maximum intensity projections (MIP) or volume-rendered images. Image quality, however, improves if contrast medium is administered since it strongly enhances the contrast to non-vascular structures. Contrast medium of course is mandatory for the diagnosis of pulmonary embolism.

MSCT will soon become the standard imaging procedure for patients with suspected pulmonary embolism, because it overcomes current limitations of spiral CT and is able to directly demonstrate even small peripheral emboli [13]. MSCT is an excellent tool to demonstrate peripheral arteriovenous malformations (AVM) and to evaluate the feeding and draining arteries with better spatial resolution than was possible with spiral CT (Fig. 4). Other congenital malformations, such as aberrant pulmonary venous return or pulmonary sling, pose no problem on MSCT.

Tracheobronchial System

MSCT has vastly improved the evaluation of the tracheobronchial system. With a high-resolution protocol, even small bronchi can be evaluated, and the differentiation between ectatic and normal bronchi is much easier. Stenoses and tumor invasion can easily be detected. Virtual bronchoscopy used to be limited to the central tracheobronchial system, but MSCT has increased spatial resolution and now allows for evaluation even of subsegmental bronchi.

Although virtual bronchoscopy yields excellent displays of the tracheobronchial system, its clinical impact has been limited. The technique is most powerful if additional display modalities (thick MPR, volume rendering, etc.) are being employed (Fig. 3). Relative to fiberoptic bronchoscopy, MSCT is much less invasive and very well tolerated by the patients. It can display the bronchial system distal to a narrow stenosis. Inversion of the viewing direction of the virtual 'bronchoscope' is possible, and one is able to look towards the proximal portions of the tracheobronchial system. Most importantly, however, is that all of the additional information from the surrounding structures is available from the scan [14]. Thus, there is information of the transmural extent of a tumor, the presence and location of lymph nodes, and the location of suspicious areas within the lung parenchyma.

Diffuse Lung Disease

Conventional (discontinuous) HRCT will remain the mainstay of evaluation for diffuse lung disease. Although MSCT of the whole lung is possible and yields excellent results, radiation exposure is still greater than with conventional HRCT. There is no data yet whether coronal sections (Fig. 2) improve diagnostic evaluation. For follow-up of patients under therapy, however, multi-slice scanning may be superior if it is performed in a discontinuous fashion, similar to conventional HRCT. With MSCT, four sections instead of only one section are obtained. Therefore, identical sections can be better reproduced.

The main advantage lies in patients in whom focal and diffuse lung disorders are suspected. Here, MSCT is able to provide both a standard CT examination and a HRCT scan (Fig. 1). This patient group includes immunocompromised patients with fever in whom a viral or fungal infection is suspected (focal or diffuse disease).

Summary

MSCT offers exciting new opportunities for imaging of the lung parenchyma. In the near future, it will become the standard procedure for most CT examinations of the lungs.

References

1. Klingenbeck-Regn K, Schaller S, Flohr T, Ohnesorge B, Kopp AF, BaumU (1999) Subsecond multi-slice computed tomography: basics and applications. Eur J Radiol 31:110–124
2. Schöpf UJ, Brüning R, Becker C, Eibel R, Hong C, von Rückmann B, Stadie A, Reiser MF (1999) Imaging of the thorax with multislice spiral CT. Radiologe 39:943–951
3. Eibel R, Brüning R, Schöpf UJ, Leimeister P, Stadie A, Reiser MF (1999) Image analysis in multislice spiral CT of the lung with MPR and MIP reconstructions. Radiologe. 39:952–957
4. Tillich M, Kammerhüber, Reittner P, et al. (1997) Detection of pulmonary nodules with helical CT: comparison of cine and film-based viewing. AJR Am J Roentgenol 169:1611–1614
5. Munden RF, Pugatch RD, Liptay MJ, Sugarbaker DJ, Le LU (1997) Small pulmonary lesions detected at CT: clinical importance. Radiology 202:105–110
6. Seemann MD, Staebler A, Beinert T, et al. (1999) Usefulness of morphological characteristics for the differentiation of benign from malignant solitary lesions using HRCT. Eur Radiol 9:409–417
7. Henschke C, McCauley D, Yankelevitz D, et al. (1999) Early lung cancer action project: overall design an findings from baseline screening. Lancet 354:99–105
8. Gdeedo A, van Schil P, Corthouts B, van Mieghem F, van Meerbeeck J, van Marck E (1997) Prospective evaluation of CT and mediastinoscopy in mediastinal lymph node staging. Eur Respir J 10:1547–1551
9. Storto ML, Ciccotosto C, Guidotti A, Merlino B, Patea RL, Bonomo L (1998) Neoplastic extension across pulmonary fissures: value of spiral CT and multiplanar reformations. J Thorac Imag 13:204–210
10. Mori K, Hirose T, Machida S, Yokoi K, Tominaga K, Moriyama N, Sasagawa M (1998) Helical CT diagnosis of pleural dissemination in lung cancer: comparison of thick section and thin section helical CT. J Thorac Imag 13:211–218
11. Shimoyama K, Murata K, Takahashi M, Morita R (1997) Pulmonary hilar lymph node metastases from lung cancer: evaluation based on morphology at thin section, incremental dynamic CT. Radiology 203:187–195
12. Nitta N, Takahashi M, Murata K, Morita R (1998) Ultra low-dose helical CT of the chest. AJR Am J Roentgenol 171:383–385
13. Remy JM, Remy J, Baghaie F, Fribourg M, Artaud D, Duhamel A (2000) Clinical value of thin collimation in the diagnostic workup of pulmonary embolism. AJR Am J Roentgenol 175:407–411
14. McAdams HP, Goodman PC, Kussin P (1998) Virtual bronchoscopy for directing transbronchial needle aspiration of hilar and mediastinal lymph nodes. AJR Am J Roentgenol 170:1361–1364

Multisclice CT in Pulmonary Embolism

U. Joseph Schoepf

Introduction

Pulmonary embolism (PE) is an elusive disease of protean nature with a high incidence and mortality. Its diagnosis remains challenging – to this day an estimated 50% of fatal cases of PE are not diagnosed antemortem [1]. Recent years have seen an increasing importance of computed tomography (CT) in the diagnosis of PE, mainly brought about by the advent of fast CT image acquisition techniques [2–4]. Competing imaging modalities are in decline: Nuclear scanning, once the first line of defense in the diagnostic algorithm of PE, is withdrawing to diagnostic niches due to limited availability and a notorious lack of specificity [5]. The one-time gold standard for the diagnosis of PE, pulmonary angiography, is becoming increasingly tarnished [6,7]. Magnetic resonance (MR) imaging may be a promising tool for the diagnosis of PE [8,9] in the future but to date has not found widespread use in emergency medicine mainly due to its long examination times and difficulties in patient monitoring. In contrast, CT has become established as a widely available [10], safe, cost-effective [11], and accurate modality for a quick and comprehensive [4,12] diagnosis of the pulmonary circulation and the deep venous system [13]. The evident advantages of CT for the diagnosis of PE have become further enhanced by the introduction of multislice CT (MSCT, Siemens SOMATOM Volume Zoom) technology. It is now feasible to acquire a 1-mm scan of the entire thorax within one breath-hold. Perceived limitations of CT for the depiction of peripheral emboli are thus overcome. In the following sections we will discuss the clinical impact of MSCT on the diagnostic algorithm of suspected PE.

Diagnosis of Pulmonary Embolism with CT – General Considerations

The most important advantage of CT over competing imaging modalities is that the mediastinal and parenchymal structures can be evaluated [4]. This makes it possible to directly visualize the embolus and the distension of the right cardiac cavities, which is a measure of the right heart load of the patient [14]. Moreover it has been shown that up to two thirds of patients with initially suspected PE receive other diagnoses [15]. With CT, potentially life-threatening, alternative causes of the clinical signs and symptoms in a patient with chest pain and a normal radiograph, such as aortic dissection, can be reliably identified. In addition, it seems to be largely unknown that CT also appears to be the diagnostic modality of choice in pregnant patients with suspected PE. Even with high scanner settings the average fetal radiation dose with CT is significantly less than nuclear perfusion lung scanning so that CT for suspected PE may even be acceptable in pregnancy [16].

In spite of these eminent advantages, a case has frequently been made against CT imaging of PE, based on its alleged lack of accuracy for peripheral emboli. The significance of such small emboli in the periphery of the lung is uncertain and will be discussed in a later section. Meanwhile, CT has demonstrated its high accuracy for the detection of PE down to the segmental arterial level [17]. Its ability to detect subsegmental emboli rivals that of invasive pulmonary arteriography: In a recent study the interobserver agreement for detection of subsegmental emboli with pulmonary angiography was a mere 66% [7]. With CT, an accuracy of the same range for the detection of subsegmental emboli could be achieved back in 1995 with a first generation spiral scanner without a subsecond image acquisition capability [17]. Thus, for diagnostic purposes there is no clinical advantage of subjecting a patient to invasive pulmonary angiography, a procedure that carries a small, but definite risk [18]. In addition, CT proved to be the most cost-effective modality in the diagnostic algorithm of PE [11], which is becoming increasingly more important in today's socio-economic environments.

Diagnosis of Pulmonary Embolism with Single-Slice CT

It could be shown that superior visualization of segmental and subsegmental pulmonary arteries can be achieved with 2-mm versus 3-mm collimation [19], probably due to reduced volume averaging and improved analysis of small-sized vessels with thinner slices. However, using single-slice CT (SCT) systems the range, which can be covered with thin collimation within one breath-hold is rather limited, even if high pitch factors are used [3,19]. For this reason we employ 3-mm collimation in order to be able to scan the entire thorax so that important differential diagnoses that cause the patient's signs and symptoms can be recognized (Table 1). In general, CT investigations for suspected PE should be performed using caudo-cranial acquisition. This reduces motion artifacts from respiration, since the caudal portions of the lung, which are most affected by respiratory motion, are scanned first. Another reason is reduction of beam hardening and streak artifacts arising from dense contrast material in the superior vena cava and subclavian vein during the early phase of contrast material injection. In addition, caudo-cranial acquisition improves vessel opacification of upper lobe arteries, which tend to be poorly opacified and thus difficult to evaluate when a cranio-caudal scan direction is used. One disadvantage of SCT is that the 0.75-s slice acquisition time is still too long to effectively reduce cardiac pulsation artifacts in the vicinity of the heart [20]. Segmental and subsegmental arteries in paracardiac lung segments thus tend to be blurred, so that definitive exclusion of isolated emboli in these vessels is not always feasible [3].

Table 1. Optimized SCT scan protocol for suspected PE

	Collimation	Table feed	Gantry rotation	Pitch	kV	mAs	Contrast volume	Flow	Delay	Recon/increm.
SCT	3 mm	8 mm/s	0.75 s	2	120	120	140 ml	4 ml/s	14 s	3/2, 5/5 (lung)

Table 2. Optimized MSCT scan protocols

	Collimation	Table feed	Gantry rotation	Pitch	kV	mAs	Contrast volume	Flow	Delay	Recon/increm
Acute PE	4x2.5 mm	30 mm/s	0.5 s	6	120	120	80 ml/120 ml (veins)	4 ml/s	18 s	3/2, 5/5 (lung)
Peripheral PE	4x1 mm	12 mm/s	0.5 s	6	120	120	120 ml	4 ml/s	18 s	1.25/1, 5/5 (lung)
PH	4x1 mm	8 mm/s	0.75 s	6	120	120	130 ml	4 ml/s	20 s	1.25/1, 5/5 (lung), 1.25/10 (HR)
ECG gating	4x2.5	Heart-rate dependent	0.5 s	Heart-rate dependent	120	240	140 ml	3.5 ml/s	16	3/2, 5/5 (lung)
Veins	4x5 mm	70 mm/s	0.5 s	7	120	120	No additional contrast	-	150 s total	5/5 delay

Diagnosis of Pulmonary Embolism with Multislice CT

Multislice CT for Imaging Acute PE

In suspected PE, both speed and attention to detail are crucial. In the emergency situation, in dyspneic or uncooperative patients the presence of central emboli (i.e., including segmental pulmonary arteries) must be verified or ruled out within few seconds. To this end we use a MSCT (Siemens SOMATOM Volume Zoom) protocol that comprises 500-ms rotation, pitch of 6, and 4 x 2.5-mm collimation (Table 2). With this protocol the entire thorax (25 cm) can be covered within 8 s. This unprecedented speed results in optimal image quality even in the most dyspneic or uncooperative individuals and represents an invaluable gain in our ability to care for critically ill patients (Figs. 1,2). If only the pulmonary vessels are to be evaluated, the amount of contrast material can be substantially reduced (Table 2), which is an important advantage in the elderly population with impaired cardiac and renal function.

Multislice CT for Imaging Peripheral Pulmonary Arteries

The clinical significance of small peripheral emboli in segmental and sub-segmental pulmonary arteries in the absence of central emboli is uncertain. It has been shown that 6% [5] to 30% [21] of patients with documented PE present with clots only in subsegmental and smaller arteries. It is assumed that one important function of the lung is to prevent small emboli from entering the arterial circulation [22]. Such emboli are thought to form even in healthy individuals although this notion has never been substantiated [23]. Controversy also exists as to whether the treatment of small emboli, once detected, may result in a better clinical outcome for patients [24,22,21,25]. There seems to be agreement, though,

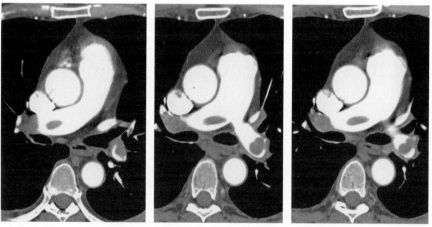

Fig. 1. Acute PE. A central saddle embolus extends into the right and left main pulmonary artery. Scan protocol: 2.5-mm collimation, pitch 6, total scan time: 8 s

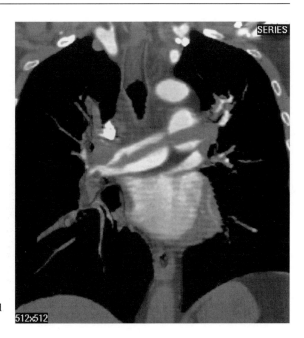

Fig. 2. Same patient as in Fig. 1. The extent of the embolus is intuitively visualized by a coronal volume rendered display

that the presence of peripheral emboli is an important indicator of current deep vein thrombosis, thus potentially heralding more severe embolic events [1,21,15]. A burden of small peripheral emboli may also have prognostic relevance in individuals with cardio-pulmonary restrictions [22,21] and for the development of chronic pulmonary hypertension in patients with thromboembolic disease [21]. Until the argument over the clinical significance of small clots is finally settled, the quest to improve the accuracy of CT for the detection of segmental and sub-segmental PE appears to be justified.

The advent of MSCT allows covering extensive volumes with thin collimation within a single breath-hold. It could be shown that superior visualization of segmental and subsegmental pulmonary arteries can be achieved with 2-mm versus 3-mm collimation [19], probably due to reduced volume averaging and improved analysis of small-sized vessels with progressively thinner slices. Use of 2-mm collimation SCT with a pitch of 2 (4-mm table-feed per 0.75-s revolution) which was proposed as the optimized acquisition protocol using SCT [19] makes it possible to cover a volume from the aortic arch to the base of the heart (10–12 cm) within 19–23 s. A 1-mm collimation MSCT acquisition with a pitch of 6 (6-mm table feed per 0.5-s revolution) covers the same range in 8–10 s (Fig. 3). Inclusion of the entire chest in the MSCT examination enhances the diagnostic value of the study, since other diseases in the periphery of the lung can also be detected. Therefore, if a meticulous analysis of peripheral pulmonary arteries for the exclusion of small clots is required, e.g., in patients with poor cardiorespiratory reserve, we cover the entire chest (25-cm) with 1-mm collimation and pitch of 6 within 20 s. Thus, despite of the use of thinner, 1-mm collimation, the acquisition speed can be significantly increased with MSCT. At the same time, the high

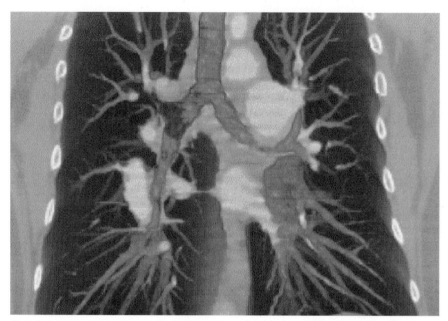

Fig. 3. Volume rendering of normal anatomy within the thoracic cavity. The quality of any kind of three-dimensional post-processing is improved by acquisition of thin slices with MSCT. Scan protocol: 1-mm collimation, pitch 6, total scan time: 22 s

spatial resolution of 1-mm sections, if read from a monitor, significantly increases the detection rate of segmental and subsegmental pulmonary emboli compared with conventional SCT (Fig. 4). This increase in the rate of detection is likely directly related to the accurate depiction, without volume averaging, of

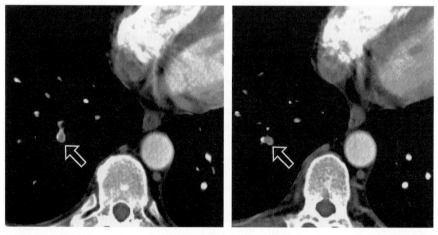

Fig. 4. Small isolated emboli in segmental and subsegmental pulmonary arteries of the right lower lobe (*arrows*). The high spatial resolution of a 1-mm collimation MSCT acquisition reduces partial volume averaging and allows reliable detection of small peripheral emboli

progressively thinner vessels by use of thinner sections. Isolated emboli in para-cardiac segmental and subsegmental arteries represent a diagnostic challenge to conventional SCT scanners [3]. Transmitted cardiac pulsation artifacts result in blurring of these vessels, even with the use of subsecond gantry rotation and 0.75-s temporal resolution. A definitive exclusion of isolated emboli is often precluded. This limitation is somewhat amenable to the faster temporal resolution of volume zoom scanning with 0.5-s gantry rotation. A more sophisticated method of improving the visualization of paracardiac lung vessels is to synchronize the scan acquisition to the ECG of the patient, in this way freezing cardiac motion and reducing transmitted pulsation artifacts [20]. With the Volume Zoom ECG software package we achieve ECG synchronization by means of retrospective cardiac gating. With retrospective ECG gating, an oversampling of data is performed by reducing the pitch. This way, axial sections can be reconstructed at arbitrary phases of the cardiac cycle. With use of partial view 240° image reconstruction, the temporal resolution of MSCT scanning can routinely be reduced to 250 ms. If image data from two consecutive heart cycles is used (biphasic reconstruction), a minimum temporal resolution of 130 ms can be achieved with some heart rates. In our preliminary experience, the visualization of paracardiac arteries can be significantly improved by using the cardiac gated technique. Thus, traditional limitations of CT for the diagnosis of small peripheral emboli appear to be overcome.

Multislice CT for Evaluating Pulmonary Hypertension

Pulmonary hypertension (PH) of the precapillary lung vasculature is a diagnostic challenge. The host of potential underlying disorders includes idiopathic disease, recurrent embolism and structural lung changes, among other more readily identifiable causes [26]. CT has traditionally been an important tool in the diagnostic algorithm of PH, allowing for an accurate assessment of both pathogenesis and extent of the disease. High resolution CT (HRCT) is the gold standard for evaluating a patient with suspected PH for structural lung changes that may cause increased pre- or postcapillary pressure within the lung vessels. Mosaic attenuation on HRCT (Fig. 5), combined with distal pruning of pulmonary arteries, is a telltale sign of impaired pulmonary perfusion due to recurrent peripheral embolism as the underlying cause. Contrast-enhanced SCT allows for direct visualization of more centrally located chronic thromboemboli (Fig. 6) and helps to determine whether the disease is amenable to surgical thrombendarterectomy. If neither structural lung changes nor signs of thromboembolism are found in the absence of other identifiable etiologies for PH, such as congenital heart disease or tumor embolism, a diagnosis of primary pulmonary hypertension (PPH) is usually considered. Since the differential diagnosis of PH includes diseases with both a focal and diffuse character, the entire pathology frequently cannot be appreciated with a single CT technique. Conventional thick collimation SCT may not suffice to assess interstitial changes. If only HRCT is performed, focal pathology, such as thromboembolism, is easily missed due to the high-frequency reconstruction algorithms and because scans are acquired at

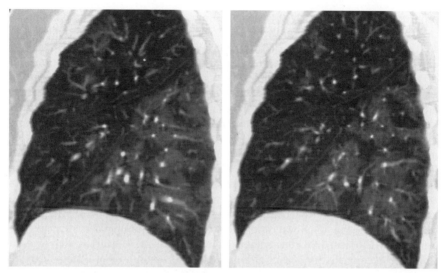

Fig. 5. Sagittal reformatting of a 1-mm collimation MSCT data set of a patient with pulmonary hypertension secondary to recurrent peripheral embolism. The distribution of the mosaic perfusion of the lung parenchyma is well visualized. Also note the clear delineation of the interlobar fissures on the reformatted sagittal image

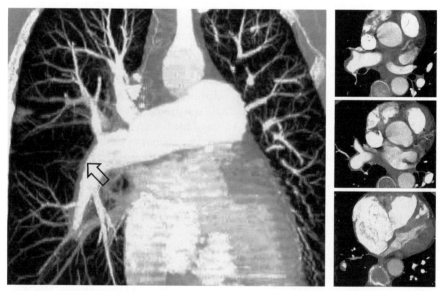

Fig. 6. Coronal MIP view and axial source images in a patient with pulmonary hypertension secondary to chronic thromboembolism. The full extent of the thrombotic wall changes is seen on the MIP view (*arrow*), which facilitates planning of thrombendarterectomy in this patient

only every 10–20 mm. In patients with suspected PH it is therefore often necessary to perform both SCT and HRCT for a comprehensive assessment of the
underlying pathology. Now, a single, breath-held, 1-mm collimation MSCT acquisition generates a set of raw data that provides all options for image reconstruction, and multiple diagnostic problems can be addressed by performing a single
contrast-enhanced scan (Table 2). In patients with suspected PH we routinely
perform a 1-mm reconstruction of the entire chest, which, if read from a monitor,
allows a highly sensitive detection of small peripheral thrombotic changes. In
addition, from the same set of raw data, 5-mm contiguous lung sections and
1-mm HRCT sections at every 1-cm are routinely performed. Thus, from a single
set of raw data a comprehensive analysis for gross and diffuse lung changes and
for thromboembolic disease becomes feasible.

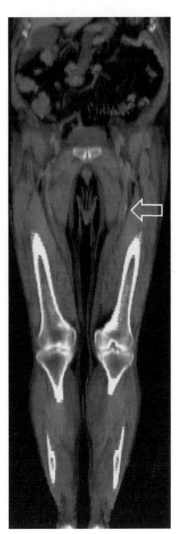

Fig. 7. Coronal volume rendered view of a patient with acute
PE and residual thrombosis in his left femoral vein (*arrow*).
A range of more than 1 m was covered in 22 s with 5-mm
collimation and a pitch of 6 with MSCT

Multislice CT for Imaging Deep Venous Thrombosis

Combined CT venography and pulmonary angiography is a diagnostic test that screens for pulmonary embolism and deep venous thrombosis (DVT) using a single contrast medium infusion. This technique has been proposed as a cost-effective means for excluding lower extremity venous thrombosis in patients undergoing CT pulmonary angiography [27]. Key advantages include the fact that no additional contrast media need to be injected to evaluate both the pulmonary vessels and the deep venous system. We use the volume covering capabilities which have become available with MSCT to establish a comprehensive diagnosis of PE and DVT in patients without a known source of emboli. In this setting, we administer a full dose of 120 cc of contrast material while scanning the pulmonary arteries and then cover the entire subphrenic venous system during venous enhancement without any additional contrast material. Using 500-ms rotation, 4x5-mm collimation and pitch 7, a 100-cm volume can be covered in less than 20 s

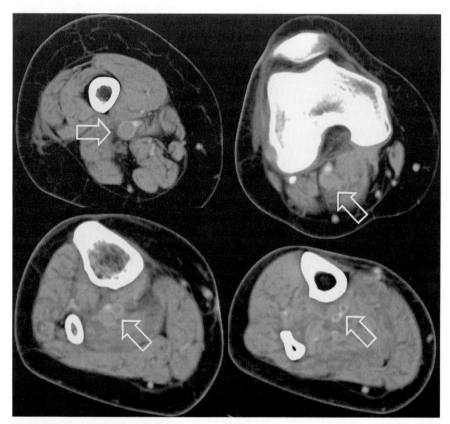

Fig. 8. A diagnosis of residual thrombosis is best made using axial source images. An MSCT scan of the lower extremity of this patient with acute PE reveals residual thrombosis in the thigh and in calve veins

(Fig. 7). In a patient with acute pulmonary embolism who is bound for the intensive care unit, a comprehensive diagnosis of the extent of thrombembolic disease, the source of emboli and potential residual thrombosis can be diagnosed in a single session by using this approach. CT may even have an advantage over Doppler sonography and conventional venography since extensive residual thrombosis in the abdominal and pelvic venous systems may be better visualized with CT. Thrombosis in the calf veins (Fig. 8) may be less accurately depicted with CT but this usually does not represent a life-threatening condition. Experience also taught us that repeated referrals for suspected malignancy as the underlying cause for PE are markedly reduced by performing combined pulmonary MSCT angiography and MSCT venography as an initial examination for suspected acute PE. Thus, using our approach time consuming and expensive additional examinations in critically ill patients can be effectively avoided.

References

1. Patriquin L, Khorasani R, Polak JF (1998) Correlation of diagnostic imaging and subsequent autopsy findings in patients with pulmonary embolism. AJR Am J Roentgenol 171:347–349
2. Remy-Jardin M, Remy J (1999) Spiral CT angiography of the pulmonary circulation. Radiology 212:615–636
3. Schoepf UJ, Helmberger T, Holzknecht N, Kang DS, Bruening RD, Aydemir S, Becker CR, Muehling O, Knez A, Haberl R, Reiser MF (2000) Segmental and subsegmental pulmonary arteries: evaluation with electron- beam versus spiral CT. Radiology 214:433–439
4. Schoepf U, Bruening R, Konschitzky H, Becker CR, Knez A, Weber J, Mueling O, Herzog P, Huber A, Haberl R, Reiser M (2000) Pulmonary embolism: comprehensive diagnosis using electron-beam computed tomography for detection of emboli and assessment of pulmonary blood flow. Radiology (in press)
5. PIOPED-Investigators (1990) Value of the ventilation / perfusion scan in acute pulmonary embolism. JAMA 95:498–502
6. Diffin D, Leyendecker JR, Johnson SP, Zucker RJ, Grebe PJ (1998) Effect of anatomic distribution of pulmonary emboli on interobserver agreement in the interpretation of pulmonary angiography. AJR Am J Roentgenol 171:1085–1089
7. Stein PD, Henry JW, Gottschalk A (1999) Reassessment of pulmonary angiography for the diagnosis of pulmonary embolism: relation of interpreter agreement to the order of the involved pulmonary arterial branch. Radiology 210:689–691
8. Meaney J, Weg JG, Chenevert TL, Stafford-Johnson D, Hamilton BH, Prince MR (1997) Diagnosis of pulmonary embolism with magnetic resonance angiography. N Engl J Med 336:1422–1427
9. Roberts DA, Gefter WB, Hirsch JA, Rizi RR, Dougherty L, Lenkinski RE, Leigh JS, Jr., Schnall MD (1999) Pulmonary perfusion: respiratory-triggered three-dimensional MR imaging with arterial spin tagging–preliminary results in healthy volunteers. Radiology 212:890–895
10. Bankier A, Herold CJ, Fleischmann D, Janata-Schwatczek K (1998) Spiral CT angiography in diagnosis of acute pulmonary embolism. What factors modify implementation of standard algorithms? Radiologe 38:248–255
11. van Erkel AR, van Rossum AB, Bloem JL, Kievit J, Pattynama PNT (1996) Spiral CT angiography for suspected pulmonary embolism: a cost-effectiveness analysis. Radiology 201:29–36
12. Schoepf UJ, Bruning RD, Becker CR, Konschitzky H, Muhling O, Stabler A, Knez A, Helmberger T, Holzknecht N, Haberl R, Reiser MF (1998) Diagnosis of pulmonary embolism with spiral and electron-beam CT. Radiologe 38:1036–1044
13. Schoepf U, R. Brüning, C. Becker, R. Eibel, C. Hong, B. von Rückmann, A. Stadie, M. F. Reiser (1999) Imaging of the thorax with multislice spiral CT. Radiologe 11: 943–951
14. Wintersperger BJ, Stabler A, Seemann M, Holzknecht N, Helmberger T, Fink U, Reiser MF (1999) Evaluation of right heart load with spiral CT in patients with acute lung embolism. Fortschr Röntgenstr 170:542–549
15. Hull R, Raskob GE, Ginsberg JS, Panju AA, Brill-Edwards P, Coates G, Pineo GF (1994) A noninvasive strategy for the treatment of patients with suspected pulmonary embolism. Arch Intern Med 154:289–297

16. Winer-Muram H, Boone JM, Tankiwale A, Lombardo GL, Russi TJ, Muram D (1999) Helical CT for pregnant patients with suspected pulmonary embolism: is it safe? Radiology 213(P):128
17. Goodman L, Curtin JJ, Mewissen MW, Foley WD, Lipchik RJ, Crain MR, Sagar KB, Collier BD (1995) Detection of pulmonary embolism in patients with unresolved clinical and scintigraphic diagnosis: helical ct versus angiography. AJR Am J Roentgenol 164:1369–1374
18. Stein PD AC, Alavi A et al (1992) Complications and validity of pulmonary angiography in acute pulmonary embolus. Circulation 85:462–468
19. Remy-Jardin M, Remy J, Artaud D, Deschildre F, Duhamel A (1997) Peripheral pulmonary arteries: optimization of the spiral CT acquisition protocol. Radiology 204:157–163
20. Schoepf UJ, Becker CR, Bruening RD, Helmberger T, Staebler A, Leimeister P, Reiser MF (1999) Electrocardiographically gated thin-section CT of the lung. Radiology 212:649–654
21. Oser RF, Zuckerman DA, Gutierrez FR, Brink JA (1996) Anatomic distribution of pulmonary emboli at pulmonary angiography: implications for cross sectional imaging. Radiology 199:31–35
22. Gurney JW (1993) No fooling around: direct visualization of pulmonary embolism. Radiology 188:618–619
23. Tetalman MR, Hoffer PB, Heck LL, Kunzmann A, Gottschalk A (1973) Perfusion lung scan in normal volunteers. Radiology 106:593–594
24. Remy-Jardin M, Remy J, Deschildre F, Artaud D, Beregi JP, Hossein-Foucher C, Marchandise X, Duhamel A (1996) Diagnosis of pulmonary embolism with spiral CT: comparison with pulmonary angiography and scintigraphy. Radiology 200:699–706
25. Novelline R, Baltarowich O, Athanasoulis C, Greenfield A, McKusick K (1978) The clinical course of patients with suspected pulmonary embolism and a negative pulmonary angiogram. Radiology 126:561–567
26. Frazier AA, Galvin JR, Franks TJ, Rosado-De-Christenson ML (2000) From the archives of the AFIP: pulmonary vasculature: hypertension and infarction. Radiographics 20:491–524
27. Loud P, Grossman CD, Klippenstein DL, Ray CE (1998) Combined CT venography and pulmonary angiography: a new diagnostic technique for suspected thrombembolic disease. AJR Am J Roentgenol 170:951–954

The Radiologist's Role in Radiation Exposure during Chest Computed Tomography

Peter Vock, Ulrike Brehmer

Stochastic somatic and genetic effects of ionising radiation exposure are recognised to be biologically significant. Effective dose is the single best parameter to estimate the biologic impact. Depending on the geographic location, natural population exposure in central Europe is estimated to be around 3 mSv/year and medical exposure 1–1.5 mSv/year (Table 1). More important, the relative contribution of 25–50% [1, 2, 3, 4] of CT to the medical exposure of the population is increasing due both to a still increasing number of studies and a decreasing contribution by non-computed tomography (CT) studies (caused by decreasing frequency and individual dose due to more and more pulsed fluoroscopy). Individual exposure through chest examinations has a wide range between around 0.05 mSv for a single posteroanterior chest radiograph and more than 20 mSv for cardiac intervention (Table 2). CT is characterised by an extra-

Table 1. Population exposure to ionising radiation (Switzerland 1994, Swiss Federal Office of Health)

Non-medical exposure:	Natural (cosmic, external, internal)	30%	1.2 mSv/y
	Radon	40%	1.6 mSv/y
	Industrial	5%	0.2 mSv/y
Medical exposure:	Non-CT	(Around 60%)	
	CT	(Around 40%[a])	1–(1.5[b]) mSv/y
Total population exposure:			4 mSv/y

[a]Relative contribution of CT to medical exposure 25% to almost 50% [1, 2, 3, 4]
[b]Estimated value for Germany 1.5 mSv/y. CT, computed tomography

Table 2. X-ray exposure through individual chest examinations. The values are approximate; they were modified from unpublished data of the Institute of Applied Radiophysics, University of Lausanne, Switzerland, 2000

Protocol	Effective dose
Standard chest CT (female>male)	~10 (3–20) mSv
Sequential (10/10,200 mA) or spiral (pitch1)	(~PET FDG)
HRCT (1/10,200mA)	~1 mSv
Chest radiography (pa/lat)	~0.15 mSv
Oesophagus contrast study	~6–7 mSv
Cardiac/coronary angiography	~8–22 mSv
PTCD	~14–29 mSv

HRCT, high resolution computed tomography; PET, positron emission tomography; FDG, fluoro-desoxy-glucose; pa, posteroanterior; lat, lateral; PTCD, percutaneous transhepatic cholangiography with drainage

ordinary medical usefulness but also a relatively high individual exposure. This fact makes it important both for the medical doctor requesting a study and the radiologist performing it to be aware of the exposure, to check for alternatives without ionising radiation and to reduce exposure during CT studies to the very minimum needed medically.

The recent exciting development of very fast CT scanners with multi-row detectors has even increased the indications, i.e. for screening, and has brought an enormous flexibility of scanning protocols. This asks for some easy method to estimate the variation of effective dose and dose to important organs with variable typical CT protocols [5]. Although recent scanners indicate physical parameters, such as the CT dose index (CTDI) and the dose–length product [6, 7], these are not directly related to the biologic impact. Organ dose might be estimated from CTDI using conversion factors [8, 9]. Based on recommendations of the International Commission on Radiation Protection (ICRP), phantom studies and computer simulation, Kalendar et al. [10] developed a software program that allows the entering of scanner-specific constants, individual protocol parameters, and the calculation of organ and effective dose (WinDose, Wellhöfer Co., D 90592 Schwarzenbruck). It was the aim of our project to estimate the exposure of important organs and the effective dose in several typical chest CT protocols in order to get an estimation of the contribution of different protocol parameters and to help design optimised CT protocols.

Materials and Methods

Using the software program of Kalender et al. [10], we calculated the organ dose to the lung, the breast and the gonads and the effective dose for seven different chest CT protocols, a general study of the isolated chest, the chest and abdomen, CT pulmonary arteriography without and with additional full chest CT and low dose protocols for high-resolution CT (HRCT) and spiral chest CT (Table 3). All values were based on ICRP 60 recommendations. Except for the general protocol used to see the difference between the two genders, values for females only were

Table 3. Protocols

	Slice	Pitch	Rotation	mA
Chest, (f)	8 mm	1.5	0.75 s	200
Chest, (m)	8 mm	1.5	0.75 s	200
Chest and abdomen (f)	8 mm	1.5	0.75 s	200
Pulmonary CTA (f)	2 mm	2	0.75 s	240
+Pre- and post chest (f)	10/2/8 mm	1.8/2/1.5	0.75 s	120/240/200
Low dose				
Sequential HRCT (f)	1 mm	Feed 10 mm	0.75 s	90
Spiral chest (f)	8 mm	2	0.75 s	90
Multi-slice chest (f)[a]	4x1 mm	1.5	0.5 s	100

[a] Simulated for multi-slice scanner based on the computed tomography dose index of Somatom Plus 4 single-slice scanner. f, female; m, male; HRCT high resolution computed tomography; CTA, computed tomography angiography

obtained. All protocols were simulated on a single-slice scanner (Somatom Plus 4) at 120 kVp, using the spiral technique except for the sequential HRCT protocol. Furthermore, using the scanner characteristics of a Somatom Plus 4, a multi-slice chest CT protocol, as used on the multi-slice scanner Somatom Plus 4 Volume Zoom, was simulated, assuming four 1-mm slices to be equivalent to one slice with a collimation of 4 mm.

Results

The effective dose of our representative protocols varied widely between 0.22 mSv and 9.49 mSv (Table 4) and was 4.22 mSv for the female standard chest CT protocol, with a significant dose around 12 mSv to the lung and the breast and a low scatter dose to the gonads. The male standard protocol, due to the difference in breast and gonad dose, had an effective dose of only 3.35 mSv. The added examination of the entire abdomen more than doubled the effective dose to 9.49 mSv and also showed a significant gonad dose of 9.1 mSv in a standard female phantom. For pulmonary CT angiography, the decreased scanning range between the top of the aortic arch and below the inferior pulmonary vein, despite a slightly increased current of 240 mA instead of 200 mA, was responsible for a reduced effective dose of 2.20 mSv. Similarly, the dose to the lung, the breast and the gonads was somewhat lower. However, when the same protocol was combined with a precontrast scan using reduced milliampage and increased pitch and a postcontrast study of the entire chest to check for alternative pathology, the effective dose rose to 8.57 mSv with a much higher dose to the lung and the breast of roughly 25 mSv each.

The two low-dose protocols studied showed much reduced exposure. Using 67.5 mA, the effective dose was 0.22 mSv for HRCT of 1-mm slices every 10 mm and 1.34 mSv for the spiral volumetric protocol. Local organ dose to the lung and the breast was roughly 3–3.5 times the effective dose. Finally, the simulated multi-slice protocol of the entire chest using 50 mA and a pitch of 1.5 was estimated to cause an effective dose of 1.35 mSv.

Table 4. Selected organ and effective dose using different chest computed tomography protocols

120 kVp, Somatom P4 protocol	Organ dose (mSv)			Effective dose (mSv)
	Lung	Breast	Gonads	
Chest (f) 8/1.5/200	11.6	12.1	0.05	4.22
Chest (m) 8/1.5/200	11.5	-	0.00	3.35
Chest and abdomen (f) 8/1.5/200	11.9	12.3	9.1	9.49
Pulmonary CTA (f) 2/2/240	7.4	10.0	0.002	2.20
+Pre- and post chest (f) 10-2-8	24.8	25.0	0.07	8.57
Low dose				
Sequential HRCT (f)	0.7	0.8	0.001	0.22
Spiral chest (f)	3.9	4.1	0.01	1.34
Multi-slice[a] (f) 4x1/1.5/100	3.7	4.0	0.003	1.35

[a] Simulated for multi-slice scanners based on the computed tomography dose index of Somatom Plus 4 single-slice scanner. f, female; m, male; HRCT, high-resolution computed tomography; CTA, computed tomography angiography

Discussion

The development and continuous improvement of CT has had an important influence on the practise of medicine in most industrialised countries, and this influence, contrary to expectations in the 1980s and 1990s, is still growing, despite the introduction of magnetic resonance imaging (MRI). New indications and an improving availability and better results with modern scanners may be the factors responsible. Parallel to the rise of the method, the contribution of CT to the medical exposure of the population has increased significantly, with official proportions of 25–40% [1, 2, 3] and, currently, close to 50%, as extrapolated in a recent publication of the Royal College of Radiologists [4]. According to the ALARA principle ("as low as reasonably achievable") of radiation protection, the medical community is responsible for an appropriate use of ionising radiation. Referring doctors are mainly requested to carefully select patients for imaging studies using ionising radiation. Sometimes no imaging test at all is needed, and sometimes ultrasound and/or MRI are appropriate alternatives. Once ionising radiation is justified, it is the radiologist's responsibility to carefully select the optimal imaging procedure and protocol, and this task has become much more challenging for CT studies than for radiography [11, 12]; this applies even more for multi-row detector CT. For the radiologist planning a CT examination, it is useful to separate the four components of radiation exposure, the localising projection view and the contribution by one tube rotation, by volume coverage and by repeated scanning (Table 5).

The localising projection scan usually provides a relatively small, although not neglectable, exposure (around 2%, [7]). Since it allows for a primary correct selection of the scan range and therefore avoids test scans, it is mostly justified. For cross-sectional imaging, the contribution by one tube rotation, i.e. one sequential scan or one subunit of a spiral scan, is the component that is most hardware dependent. The geometry of the scanner, the specific performance of the generator and the tube, filtration and the detection and conversion efficiency

Table 5. Radiation exposure components in computed tomography

Localiser (scout, topogram)
Exposure per tube rotation (one sequential scan, one subunit of spiral scan)
kVp, mA
Tube performance, filtration, scanner geometry (distances, fan)
Adaptation to patient habitus, child, ap-lat. dose modulation, organ (lung)
Detectors: geometric, quantum detection and conversion efficiency
Volume coverage (z-axis)
Sequential (overlap) – spiral (pitch) – multi-slice
Repeated scanning of identical volume
Native and IV contrast-enhanced scans, contrast bolus tagging
Dynamic enhancement: arterial/parenchymal/venous phase
Functional inspiratory and expiratory scans (air trapping)
Positional changes (gravitation, supine/prone, subpleural lines)
CT-guided biopsy/intervention (CT fluoroscopy)
Thick slice overview, subsequent thin (1–5 mm) collimation

CT, computed tomography; IV intravenous

of the data acquisition system are usually constant parameters that cannot be influenced by the radiologist. Nevertheless, appropriate selection of kVp, mA, rotation time and slice collimation is the key factor for optimal image quality at the minimal exposure. This is most extremely demonstrated by the difference of effective dose during a standard spiral chest scan in a female patient (4.22 mSv) and the corresponding value of 1.34 mSv in the low dose protocol. It is a fact common to all types of digital X-ray imaging that – in contrast to the black film seen in analogue techniques – overexposure is not easily detected by the human eye since it will just increase the signal to noise ratio (S/N) and still provide good grey scale contrast. The radiologist therefore has to adapt milliamps per rotation to the habitus and anatomical area of the patient based on the fact that – for maintaining an identical S/N – the exposure can be reduced to approximately 50% with every 4 cm of decrease of patient diameter [13]. This means reduced milliampage in children and slim patients but increased milliampages in obese patients.

Where X-ray absorption is significantly different in the anteroposterior (ap) and the lateral projection, such as for the shoulder girdle, dose modulation during one tube rotation is an excellent feature to decrease the exposure by up to 30% at an unchanged S/N. This may be done based on two orthogonal localising scans or interactively, using the absorption information of the prior rotation to select the milliamp value for the next rotation. For high-contrast organs, such as the lung and bone, milliamps can be reduced at no cost, whereas tissues and pathology with low contrast need higher milliamps. In the chest, as long as the lung is the main target, low dose protocols have been proposed in recent years and are used successfully for metastatic nodule detection and lung cancer screening [14].

The favoured voltage is still 120 kVp, and it is sometimes increased to around 140 kVp in case of increased absorption by large patient diameters or bone; scatter is increasing, whereas at low voltage, better contrast is counterbalanced by a higher percentage of low energy photons contributing to exposure but not to image formation. Thus, currently low kV protocols (80–100 kVp) are rarely used.

In order to reduce motion artefacts, the rotation time for chest studies is usually the minimum available for the scanner. Partial scans may sometimes further decrease motion within an image, but this may be paid for by a reduced image quality due to the reduced number of projections. Finally, slice collimation mainly depends on the z-axis resolution and avoidance of partial volume is needed; thinner collimation will require an increase of milliamps to maintain the S/N and will, of course, influence the solution for volume coverage. Recent multi-slice CT scanners use adaptive z-axis filtering to reduce noise and, therefore, to obtain an equal image quality at reduced milliamps.

The contribution to exposure by the type of volume coverage is different for sequential and for spiral volumetric scanning. As long as a representative sample of an organ can be obtained from systematic scanning of a small percentage of its volume, the sequential technique is definitely the best solution to keep exposure low. Unless information on topographic relation is needed, HRCT of the lung, using 1-mm slices spaced by 10 mm, is therefore the favoured technique to investigate diffuse, mostly infiltrative lung disease. Selecting all other parameters identical, exposure is 10% of the previous standard sequential protocol of obtaining contiguous 10-mm scans. Combining sequential selective sampling with a low dose protocol, we estimated an effective dose of 0.22 mSv compared with 1.34 mSv using the spiral low dose protocol.

Spiral scanning starts to be of interest as soon as gapless coverage of the z-axis is requested, as is the case for most oncologic, inflammatory and traumatic disorders. Although there is a small increase in dose by the projections outside the scanning volume needed for interpolation, increasing the pitch (p) is an excellent tool to decrease exposure at essentially no cost. The p is defined as the relation between the table feed per rotation (t) and the simultaneous beam collimation (N.c), where N is the number of detector arrays read separately and c is the thickness of one of these detector arrays. The formula $p=t/N.c$ applies. Based on a relative dose of 100% for contiguous sequential scans and roughly the same for spiral scanning at the pitch of 1, exposure is divided by p when the p is above one. Reasonable p values are between 1.5 and 2 for single-slice scanners, meaning a reduction of exposure by 33% and 50%, respectively. An increase of the pitch in addition to the reduced scan range was primarily responsible for the lower effective dose of the protocol for pulmonary CT angiography (2.20 mSv), as related to the standard chest protocol (4.22 mSv). The difference between sequential and spiral scanning is even more significant when overlapping images are used to improve z-axis resolution.

For overlapping sequential scans of 3 mm, each spaced by 2 mm, a relative exposure of 150% results, whereas overlapping images can be reconstructed from spiral raw data at the same exposure of 100% (p=1), 67% (p=1.5) or even 50% (p=2). The maximum pitch suggested currently for multi-slice scanners with four simultaneously read slices is usually 1.5 and, for better resolution, a pitch of 0.75–1 is often used. The duration of the scan is less critical despite thinner collimation, and since z-axis filtering helps reduce milliampage, exposure is usually identical or lower than in single-slice CT despite a lower pitch factor. In conclusion, when using single-slice scanners, the best solution is to choose a thin slice and a maximal pitch. Despite the consecutive degradation of the slice profile, one usually gets enough resolution at a decreased exposure.

Repeated scanning of the same anatomical area, the fourth component of exposure, is completely under the control of the radiologist, and the complexity of this task has increased recently since today's fast scanners are no longer limiting multi-phase and functional protocols. Table 5 gives some of the many reasons for repeated scanning of the same anatomical area. Precontrast-enhanced scans may be justified, where the density (for fresh blood, tiny calcifications vs vessels) or quantitation of enhancement is important, such as for solitary pulmonary nodules or tumours. Timing of scanning during and after fast intravenous bolus contrast enhancement is critical; e.g. peak pulmonary arterial, systemic arterial, venous and lesion enhancement follow each other.

To know the dynamic behaviour, more than one phase is needed and, even for one single phase, it is not easy to predict the best time. A test bolus, which means additional exposure, is therefore often used. Similarly, although it avoids an additional dose of contrast agent, contrast bolus tagging is based on repeated early low dose scans to detect the moment when a selected region of interest has reached the density threshold used to start the diagnostic scan. In the chest, functional imaging in prone position or expiration to detect atelectasis or air trapping, respectively, requires exposure in addition to the standard scanning in supine inspiration. Usually, a few sequential scans will provide this information. CT-guided biopsy and intervention cannot avoid repeated exposure to the same area but are usually justified by their unique contribution to patient management.

Our results with the pulmonary embolism protocols clearly demonstrate the significant increase of exposure to an assumed maximum of 8.57 mSv with repeated scanning. If we can restrict the study to the arterial phase protocol, the estimated exposure of 2.2 mSv can be justified even in young patients in view of the high morbidity of pulmonary embolism. In contrast, additional pre-contrast and post-contrast scans of the chest to rule out other pathology may nearly quadruple the exposure.

With single-slice scanners, the need to cover the entire chest usually requires rather thick slices of 5–10 mm; suspicious areas often then need additional thin scans of a selected subvolume. This means repeated scanning, such as the decision to add HRCT for parenchymal details to a spiral chest study. The additional exposure can be avoided with multi-slice scanners by performing one complete chest study using 1–2 mm collimation. From the raw data, without any additional exposure, both HRCT images and 5-mm thick slices can then be calculated using the axial, coronal or even sagittal plane. Aside from this significant difference in the need for repeated scans, single-slice and multi-slice scanners, as long as the same parameters are used, provide a nearly identical effective dose [15].

Our results, of course, have to be transposed with caution to clinical scanning. The simulation based on phantom measurements and calculation will never reflect the specific condition of the individual patient nor her or his habitus. Protocol simulation using a software to predict organ dose and effective dose allows for a good relative comparison of different protocols and therefore for selecting the optimal parameters for a specific clinical situation. Furthermore, consideration of age and the severity of the diagnosis in question are factors that influence protocol selection more than organ dose and effective dose of a protocol. Life-threatening conditions and studies in elderly patients render this consideration rather marginal, whereas in children or in volunteers undergoing a scientific protocol, the importance of radioprotection is even accentuated.

In conclusion, the radiologist has an increasingly important role in tailoring chest CT protocols according to the specific clinical question. A simulation software, such as the one used in this project, can easily help estimate organ and effective dose and therefore optimise protocols to the best individual use.

References

1. Jung H (1995) Strahlenrisiko: widersprüchliche angaben verunsichern öffentlichkeit und patienten. Deutsche Röntgengesellschaft: Informationen 3
2. Shrimpton PC, Wall BF (1995) The increasing importance of X-ray computed tomography as a source of medical exposure. Radiat Prot Dosim 57:413–415

3. Kaul A, Bauer J, Bernhardt D, Nosske D, Veit R (1997) Effective doses to members of the public from the diagnostic application of the ionizing radiation in Germany. Eur Radiol 7:1127–1132
4. Dixon A (ed) (1998) RCR Guidelines Working Party, 4th edn. Making the best use of a Department of Clinical Radiology. Royal College of Radiologists, p 14
5. Lenzen H, Roos N, Diederich S, Meier N (1996) Strahlenexposition bei der niedrigdosiscomputer-tomographie des thorax. Radiologe 36:483–488
6. Heinz-Peer G, Weninger F, Nowotny R, Herold CJ (1996) Strahlendosis der verschiedenen CT-verfahren in der lungendiagnostik. Radiologe 36:470–474
7. Poletti JL (1996) Patient doses from CT in New Zealand and a simple method for estimating effective dose. Br J Radiol 69:432–436
8. Geleijns J, van Unnik JG, Zoetelief J, Zweers D, Broerse JJ (1994) Comparison of two methods for assessing patient dose from computed tomography. Br J Radiol 67:360–365
9. Jones DG, Shrimpton PC (1991) Survey of CT practice in the UK. Part 3: normalised organ doses calculated using Monte Carlo techniques (NRPB-R250). National Radiological Protection Board, Chilton, UK
10. Kalender WA, Schmidt B, Zankl M, Schmidt M (1999) A PC program for estimating organ dose and effective dose values in computed tomography. Eur Radiol 9:555–562
11. Mini RL, Vock P, Müry R, Schneeberger PP (1995) Radiation exposure of patients who undergo CT of the trunk. Radiology 195:557–562
12. Wade JP, Weyman JC, Goldstone KE (1997) CT standard protocols are of limited value in assessing actual patient dose. Br J Radiol 70:1146–1151
13. Rothenberg LN, Pentlow KS (1992) AAPM tutorial: radiation dose in CT. Radiographics 12:1225–1243
14. Diederich S, Lenzen H, Windmann R, Puskas Z, Yelbuz TM, Henneken S, Klaiber T, Eameri M, Roos N, Peters PE (1999) Pulmonary nodules: experimental and clinical studies at low-dose CT. Radiology 213 (P):289–298
15. Schöpf UO, Becker CR, Bruening RD, Huber AM, Hong C, Reiser MF (1999) Multidetector-array spiral CT imaging of focal and diffuse lung disease: thin-collimation data acquisition with reconstruction of contiguous and HRCT sections. Radiology 213 (P):259

V Multislice Computed Tomography Applications in the Abdomen

Multidetector, Multislice Spiral Computed Tomography of the Abdomen: Quo Vadis

New Modes of Image Interpretation

Mark E. Baker, Brian R. Herts, William T. Davros

Sections of Abdominal Imaging and Medical Physics

The traditional approach of radiology image "interpretation" involves the following steps:
1. Recognizing normal anatomy and normal variation
2. Disease detection
3. Disease characterization into benign or malignant categories and if possible a more specific disease diagnosis
4. Disease description, including disease extent, progression, and response to therapy

Traditional radiologic investigations have paralleled these approaches to "interpretation" and seek to improve the ability to detect and characterize disease. Recently, imaging investigations have attempted to determine cost effectiveness and benefit. With computed tomography (CT), such methods of improving sensitivity and specificity have included investigations into contrast media injection, both volume and dose, and methods of delivery. Technical alterations, such as changing X-ray beam collimation, pitch, and Z-axis reconstruction interval, have all attempted to improve disease detection with spiral CT. Innumerable investigations, especially in the liver, have attempted to characterize common benign neoplasms, such as a cavernous hemangioma, in an attempt to distinguish these findings from malignancy, most commonly metastatic disease.

The traditional product of a radiology interpretation includes technique description, radiographic findings, including pertinent positives and negatives, and some form of a conclusion or impression that is a synthesis of the findings and response to the clinical question or questions. Traditionally, image interpretation has been primarily film-based, utilizing preset, default window, and level settings to assess the lung parenchyma, the liver, the kidneys, and bone. Paper or caliper measurements are used to quantify disease in an attempt to assess disease progression or regression. Regions of interest, relative to cyst enhancement, have been performed at the operator console.

Over the last 5 years, more and more imaging, particularly CT, magnetic resonance imaging (MRI), and ultrasound, has been interpreted on workstations (at the clinic, we have not read hard copy film of CT or MRI for 8 years). With spiral CT, this interpretation has been performed in the axial plane, because this is the traditional mode of image reconstruction. Initially, reading on a workstation started with the method of a single mouse click and read using a four-on-one format (monitor size 1024 x 1024 matrix), with slow progression through the study, similar to reading films. Currently, all of the CT readers at the clinic use a mouse-driven, manual cine method, with a one-on-one image format, especially in comparison with a prior imaging study. We all manually page up and down through a study, moving from the most recent study to the prior comparison study. In addition to preset window and leveling, manual windowing and leveling of the images occurs routinely. The physician on the workstation performs regions of interest and measurements.

With the advent of multi-detector, multi-slice CT, I see the following evolving methods of image "interpretation":

1. Standard multi-planar reformation (MPR) using coronal-, sagittal-, and even-curved planes. We are currently evolving our method of image reconstruction and are routinely reconstructing SOMATOM Volume Zoom abdomen images using coronal MPRs, in addition to the axial images (see below). Additionally, in the next 5 years, with developing workstations and hardware/software development, I see real-time, three-dimensional (3D) volume rendering as a potential and viable method of image interpretation. This will lead to an entirely different image product.
2. Therapy guidance using real-time, 3-D volume rendering.

We are currently scanning our patients with the SOMATOM Volume Zoom using the following technique:
  120 kVP
  120–150 mAs/reconstructed image
  Pitch 4–6
  2-mm axial image reconstruction
  3-mm coronal image reconstruction

We have found anecdotally that a coronal reconstruction of thin axial images portrays the adrenals and kidneys more effectively, especially for urologists. Further subdiaphragmatic and bowel abnormalities are often better identified. Lastly, both internist and surgeon alike "see" abnormalities better with a different perspective. We are currently comparing axial with coronal reconstructions to determine their diagnostic equivalence in disease detection.

Therapy guidance is primarily a surgical issue; however, radiation oncologists will probably also benefit. This includes not only disease detection, but also a road map vis-a-vis new modes of intervention, primarily laparoscopic. In these cases, a road map of the relational information is essential. This is important for both pre- and peri-surgical planning. Issues such as port placement and the identification of important vital structures adjacent to an abnormality are important aspects of conveying this relational information. Lastly, more and more, imaging guides the specific surgical approach.

To date, our longest experience with therapy guidance has been with urologic cases. Such areas of emerging markets in urology include ureteropelvic junction (UPJ) obstruction therapy guidance (open vs endoluminal) and laparoscopic living related donor nephrectomies. In these areas, the number and location of renal arteries, the presence and location of lumbar or gonadal veins, and the variation of renal veins, including branch fusion, are important. In addition to urologic cases, we are beginning to evaluate potential cadidates for living related liver transplants. Imaging provides important information, including hepatic venous anatomic variation, the portal vein anatomy, and hepatic arterial supply.

However, the area that we have developed the most in pre- and peri-surgical planning has been with nephron-sparing procedures. Over the last 5–8 years, nephron-sparing surgery, or so-called partial nephrectomies, has developed as the standard management strategy for the treatment of localized renal cell carcinoma, especially when renal functional preservation is desired or necessary. Many centers, including The Cleveland Clinic, have expanded the indications for this surgery and are now performing partial nephrectomies in patients with a normal contralateral kidney where there is no history of medical or urologic disease compromising renal function. Nephron-sparing surgery, regardless of the indication, remains more technically challenging than the radical nephrectomy. There is increased risk of urinary fistulas and urinomas, renal failure, postoperative hemorrhage, post operative abscess, and arterial and venous thrombosis.

At The Cleveland Clinic in the past, preoperative renal venography and arteriography, and a preoperative CT scan were performed to assess the feasibility and approach for nephron-sparing surgery. Arteriography provided a vascular road map to determine the segmental vessel(s) supplying the tumor and the other segmental vessels supplying the normal renal parenchyma. Because segmental branches of the renal artery are end arteries, there is no collateral flow between parenchyma supplied by different segmental vessels. Segmental arteries that do not supply the tumor can be injured during partial nephrectomies. Therefore, their location and aberrant origin in relation to the tumor is essential in presurgical planning. This is particularly helpful with more centrally located tumors or tumors that are deep in the kidney. Assessment of the renal venous drainage system is less important, because there is extensive collateral venous blood supply within the kidney. It is important, however, to exclude tumor involvement of the main renal veins.

The operative approach to nephron-sparing surgery starts with optimal exposure of the kidney. In general, our urologists use an extraperitoneal flank incision through the 11th and 12th rib but occasionally use a thoracoabdominal incision for very large tumors, especially those involving the upper portion of the kidney. Once the kidney is mobilized within the perirenal fascia, the perirenal fat around the tumor and the kidney are removed. In most cases, the renal artery is occluded. During renal artery occlusion, hypothermia with an ice slush bath is used to reduce ischemic injury. This approach allows for up to 3 h of safe ischemic time.

There are a variety of techniques used to perform partial nephrectomies, including apical or basilar polar segmental nephrectomies, wedge resections, and transverse resections. The vessels must be controlled, ischemic injury must be avoided, the tumor must be completely resected, the collecting system must be closed completely, hemostasis must be obtained, and the renal defect is closed with fat.

Over the last two and a half years, we have developed a 3D volume-rendered CT approach in the preoperative and intraoperative evaluation of patients undergoing nephron-sparing surgery. In a series of 97 masses in 60 patients, 3D volume rendering was successful in all patients. Of the 77 renal arteries identified at surgery, 74 were detected using 3D volume-rendered CT. CT missed three small accessory arteries, including one in a cross-fused ectopic kidney. All major venous branches in venous variants were identified. There were 69 renal veins identified at surgery, and the volume-rendered approach detected 64. The five renal veins missed when using CT were small, short, duplicated branches of the right main renal vein.

For patients undergoing a 3D volume-rendered CT, we perform a three-phase study:

1. A precontrast examination (not essential for presurgical planning, but used for mass characterization)
2. An arterial phase examination to assess the segmental arterial supply of the tumor, the vascular anatomy of the entire kidney, and the relationship of the tumor to the arteries
3. A parenchymal phase examination showing the relationship of the tumor to the collecting system, the central sinus fat, and the veins

The following protocol was used on a Plus 4, single detector/slice scanner before we installed the multidetector/slice volume zoom scanner:

Plus-4 (single-detector/slice) Nephron-Sparing Protocol

Non-Contrast
   120 kVp/200–240 mA
   750 ms
   5-mm Collimation
   Pitch 1
   5-mm Image reconstruction, every 2.5 mm
   Full field of view (FOV)

Arterial Phase
   120 kVp/240–280 mA
   750 ms
   3-mm Collimation
   Pitch 1.5–2 (depending upon patient size and necessity for increasing dose; tube mA increased for larger patients; in order to achieve Z coverage with adequate mAs/slice, the pitch is increased up to two, because there are tube heat capacity limitations)
   Keep scanning time <30 s
   Nonionic contrast media: 60% injected at 4 ml/s
   Timing bolus or bolus tracking used to estimate start scan time
   3-mm Image reconstruction, every 1.5 mm
   30 cm FOV (include kidneys and aorta)

Parenchymal Phase
    120 kVp/240 mA (mA same as precontrast)
    750 ms
    5-mm Collimation
    Pitch 1
    5-mm Image reconstruction, every 2.5 mm
    Full FOV
    Start scan 90 s after start of bolus

The arterial and parenchymal phase images are used to create a real time volume-rendered 3D model. We use either a Silicon Graphics, Inc, Onyx workstation with IPDoc software (Advanced Medical Imaging Lab, Johns Hopkins Hospital, Baltimore, Md.) or a Siemens workstation (3DVirtuoso) using a Silicon Graphics O2 workstation (incorporates the IPDoc software). For use with the workstation, a targeted reconstruction of the arterial phase images of the affected renal unit is used to maximize vascular enhancement. The precontrast and parenchymal phases are not targeted on reconstruction. Using the workstation, a 3–5 min videotape from the 3D volume rendering is made and consists of four separate portions:

1. An overall view of the kidney, demonstrating location in the retroperitoneum relative to rib cage, spine, and iliac crest.
2. The tumor is identified and, using cutting planes from anterior and flank approaches, the location and depth of each tumor is shown.
3. The relationship of the tumor to the collecting system and ureter is shown.
4. The main renal artery and vein, segmental arterial branches and any accessory vessels (including all anatomic variants) are shown. If possible, the segmental artery supplying the tumor is also demonstrated.

The format for the short videotape was defined by a close interaction between the urologic surgeon and the radiologist over an approximately 12-month period of time. This required close consultation both before and during surgery in order for the radiologist to understand the important issues in nephron-sparing surgery. Initially, longer videotapes were created. However, we now have a product that is predefined and is acceptable to the urologic surgeon. Using current software and hardware, it takes an experienced operator approximately 10–15 min to produce the videotape.

The main problem we have encountered with this protocol has been maintaining an appropriate level of arterial enhancement during a complete arterial phase spiral scan (Fig. 1a). Even with 3-mm collimation, pitch 2, using 750 ms tube rotation, we cover only 8 mm/s (with pitch 1.5, the coverage is only 6 mm/s). Generally, the Z coverage is approximately 20 cm (scanning from the top of the kidney to the aortic bifurcation in order to identify all variant arteries). In general, 20 s of scanning time is necessary in order to maintain adequate arterial enhancement. With single detector scanning, using 750 ms tube rotation, 3-mm collimation at even pitch 2, it takes 25 s to scan (6 mm/750 ms=8 mm/s; 20 cm Z coverage=25 s).

Additionally, 3-mm images tend to blur small vessels even with the forgiving volume-rendered software that we use. Despite this, we see three of the four segmental arteries over 90% of the time (anterior, posterior, apical, and basilar). The

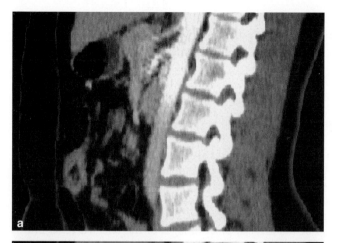

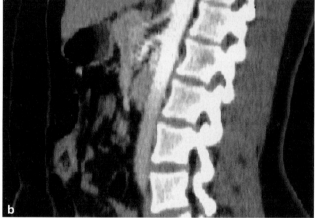

Fig. 1a, b. Volume rendered sagittal aorta derived from a Plus-4, single detector/slice scanner (a) and a SOMATOM Volume Zoom, multidetector/slice scanner (B). The aortic opacification is maintained throughout the 20 s multislice scan (b). However, with the single slice scan of 25 s, opacification progressively decreases in the inferior portion of the aorta

last problem we have encountered using the single slice scanner has been with scan misregistration. Patients are often unable to suspend respiration for more than 20 s. After 20 s, some of our patients begin to breathe, causing misregistration on the volume-rendered images (Fig. 2). Despite these problems, no diagnostic arteriograms have been performed on these patients in over 1 year. All partial nephrectomy patients are scanned in this manner and have a videotape made prior to surgery.

With the introduction of the SOMATOM Volume Zoom, Siemens, multislice CT scanner, the following protocol was developed for these patients:

SOMATOM Volume Zoom (multi-detector/slice) Nephron-Sparing Protocol

Precontrast
120 kVp/ 200–260 mAs/slice
500 ms

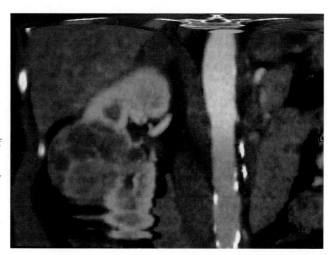

Fig. 2. Volume rendered coronal right kidney derived from a Plus-4, single detector/slice scanner. The scan time of 25 s is too long for the patient to suspend respiration. Motion secondary to breathing causes misregistration artifact in the inferior aspect of the kidney. Note the suboptimal opacification in the inferior abdominal aorta

2.5-mm Collimation
Pitch 4–5
5-mm Images, reconstruct every 2.5 mm

Arterial Phase (Alternative 1)
120 kVp/200–260 mAs/slice
500 ms
1-mm Collimation
Pitch 4–5 (pitch adjusted for Z coverage desired in 20 s)
1.5-mm Images, reconstruct every 1.5-mm and 5-mm images, reconstruct every 2.5 mm
1.5-mm Images for 3D real time volume-rendered video and 5-mm slices for interpretation

Parenchymal Phase
120 kVp/200–260 mAs/slice
500 ms
2.5-mm Collimation
Pitch 4–5
3-mm Images, reconstruct every 1.5-mm and 5-mm images, reconstruct every 2.5 mm
3-mm Slices for 3D real time volume-rendered video and 5-mm slices for interpretation

What has the multislice technology added to the evaluation of these patients? In short, the Z coverage per unit time relative to arterial opacification is excellent and much improved over the single detector/slice scanner. When the Plus 4 scans are compared with the SOMATOM Volume Zoom scans, even the distal aorta and proximal common iliac arteries are well opacified with the volume zoom technology and are suboptimal with the Plus 4 technology (Fig. 1b). We recently compared 34 patients evaluated with the multislice detector, with 33 patients using a single slice detector, evaluated for either a potential renal transplant donor or prior to a partial nephrectomy. At 6 cm from the start of the scan, using the multislice technology, the aorta was 86% of peak aortic enhancement, while with the single row detector, the aorta was only 82% of peak aortic enhancement. With the multi-slice scanner, at 10 cm from the start of the examination, the aortic enhancement was still 86% of peak aortic enhancement, whereas with the single row detector, it was only 62% of peak aortic enhancement. Therefore, the distal aorta remains optimally opacified with the multislice scanner but suboptimally with the single slice scanner. There is less misregistration artifact, because patients only need to suspend respiration for 20 s or less. Additionally, we can now scan with much narrower collimation, 1 mm, and reconstruct at 1.5 mm, giving us much better volume-rendered images and smaller vessel identification.

What is the economic impact of volume-rendered CT? Since the start of this program over 2-years ago, we have evaluated well over 300 patients for partial nephrectomies. What about other markets? In the year 2000 at The Cleveland Clinic, we have a goal to perform 150 renal transplants. Fifty of these will need to be living related donors. We estimate that 70–80 evaluations are needed for 50 such living related donor patients. Lastly, we are currently developing a living related donor, liver transplant program. To date, we have already evaluated 10 patients, and this program will only increase. As the "post-processing" program develops, more markets will emerge. While this market remains small relative to our traditional, core business of disease detection, characterization, and description, it can only grow, further enhancing CT's role in medical care.

What are the current challenges for the radiologist and the CT manufacturer? We need to define and understand the new markets for multislice CT. This includes not only presurgical planning, but also screening for diseases, such as coronary artery disease, lung cancer, and colorectal cancer. We need to think past traditional image interpretation as our product. One method of identifying new markets and products is with customer focus groups. This will not necessarily occur using a standard approach used in business. Ad hoc, informal focus groups occur in clinics, attending clinical conferences, and going to the operating room. We need to listen to the clinical needs that go beyond disease detection, characterization, and description. We also need to get clinicians to think past our traditional approaches. This will require taking risks with potential means of data portrayal.

Manufacturers will need to develop new ways of "image reconstruction." This will require some form of volume rendering that is easy and preset. It also may require development of raw data storage or volume storage, storage techniques that currently do not exist. Such volume reconstruction may be akin to multiplanar reconstruction. Lastly, and probably most importantly, we need to lobby payers for monetary reimbursement. Currently, the current procedural terminology (CPT) code for 3D CT reimburses only approximately $25 for our efforts. There is no CPT code for the information provided by real-time volume-rendered videotapes.

Suggested Reading

1. Campbell SC, Novick AC (1995) Surgical technique and morbidity of elective partial nephrectomy. Semin Urol Oncol 13:281–287
2. Hafez KS, Novick AC, Butler BP (1998) Management of small solitary unilateral renal cell carcinomas: impact of central versus peripheral tumor location. J Urol 159:1156–1160
3. Novick AC (1998) Anatomic approaches in nephron-sparing surgery for renal cell carcinoma. Atlas Urol Clin North Am 6:39–50
4. Herts BR (1998) Helical CT and CT angiography for the identification of crossing vessels at the ureteropelvic junction. Urol Clin North Am 25:259–269
5. Coll DM, Uzzo RG, Herts BR, Davros WJ, Wirth SL, Novick AC (1999) 3-Dimensional volume-rendered computerized tomography for preoperative evaluation and intraoperative treatment of patients undergoing nephron sparing surgery. J Urol 161:1097–1102
6. Herts BR, Coll DM, Lieber ML, Streem SB, Novick AC (1999) Triphasic helical CT of the kidneys: contribution of vascular phase scanning in patients before urologic surgery. AJR Am J Roentgenol 173:1273–1277
7. Coll DM, Herts BR, Davros WJ, Uzzo RG, Novick AC (2000) Preoperative use of 3D volume rendering to demonstrate renal tumors and renal anatomy. Radiographics 20:431–451

Multislice Computed Tomography of the Urinary Tract

Stuart G. Silverman

Introduction

With the advent of slip ring technology and the introduction of spiral (helical) computed tomography (CT) [1], the decade of the 1990s saw CT's role in imaging the urinary tract expand. Now, with the introduction of multi-detector technology, CT will become an even more important imaging tool in the urinary tract [2]. Multi-detector technology gives CT scanners the capability of creating four slices per gantry rotation. The four slices are derived from four channels of data, which emanate from an array of multiple detectors; the number of which depends on the manufacturer. Therefore, relative to single-slice CT (SCT), multislice CT (MSCT) results in a four-fold increase in data per gantry revolution. This results in four main advantages. The first is speed, because there is a four-fold increase in speed relative to SCT. Some manufacturers utilize two gantry rotations per second. This results in an eight-fold increase in speed. The second main advantage is that MSCT scanners allow us to obtain images over a larger area with thin collimation. This results in improved spatial resolution, not only in the z-axis with reconstructed slice thicknesses as low as 0.5 mm but near isotropic resolution in non-axial planes. The third advantage relates to scan volume. These scanners can scan larger volumes during a single breath hold, with the ability to scan from head to toe in a matter of seconds. The fourth, and perhaps most important advantage, is the flexibility provided both in acquisition protocols and in reconstruction algorithms. The radiologist has multiple options to choose from when designing CT protocols. Acquisition parameters radiologists must consider include collimation, rotation speed, pitch, and dose. Concerning reconstruction options, unlike SCT, image data sets with variable slice thicknesses can be obtained, so long as the thickness is not less than the collimation. For example, data acquisition can be formed with 1-mm collimation (or four 1-mm slices per gantry rotation) and reconstructed using both 1-mm and 2.5-mm slices or, data acquisition can be formed with 2.5-mm collimation (or four 2.5-mm slices per gantry rotation) and reconstructed using both 2.5-mm and 5-mm slices. The thin slice data can be used subsequently for multi-planar reconstruction, and the thicker slices can be viewed axially.

As a result of these technologic advances, MSCT impacts radiologic practice in several ways. First, we are no longer limited to and dependent on viewing only axial slices; sagittal and coronal images can be viewed almost immediately. Workstations allow three-dimensional (3D) views to be obtained in a matter of minutes. Second, because of the large number of images that are created, film is no longer a practical way to view studies; soft copy reading is essential. Third, when viewing axially, stack mode (1-on-1) cine viewing is the only practical way to view literally hundreds of axial images that are created by these scanners. Fourth, as some MSCT studies may yield a thousand images, data overload will tax our ability to transfer, store, and visually process large amounts of data.

These technologic advances could have a significant impact on imaging of the urinary tract. Particularly exciting applications include aiding in the evaluation of hematuria and refining further our ability to detect and characterize renal masses. Although not discussed here, other areas that are likely to be improved include the CT angiographic evaluation of the renal artery and its branches, the CT evaluation of patients after trauma, and the evaluation of patients needing nephron-sparing surgery.

Hematuria

Since its introduction in 1929, intravenous urography (IVU) has been used often as the initial test in the evaluation of patients with hematuria. In addition to being relatively safe, quick, and inexpensive, IVU has been used for many years because it is the only imaging test which provides an anatomic assessment of every major anatomic portion of the urinary tract (kidneys, intrarenal collecting system, ureters, and bladder) along with an assessment of differential function. However, IVU is often followed by cystoscopy because of its insensitivity to bladder cancer [3]. IVU has been criticized for its low yield for a variety of other disorders also [4, 5, 6]. With the advent of ultrasound and CT in the 1970s, IVU was shown to be relatively insensitive for small renal masses and incapable of being used alone to confirm that renal masses were benign [7]. The era of the 1980s and 1990s yielded many studies which showed that CT (using conventional, non-spiral technology) was the best method for detecting and characterizing renal masses [8, 9, 10], diagnosing renal injuries following trauma [11, 12, 13], and assessing patients with suspected renal infection [14]. With the introduction of spiral CT in the 1990s, CT was shown to improve further the detection and characterization of renal masses [15, 16] and the identification of urinary calculi and urinary obstruction [17]. Spiral CT was shown to delineate renal vascular anatomy both in evaluating patients for renal artery stenosis [18] and for potential renal donation [19]. Also, spiral CT has been proposed as a potential method to evaluate the urinary bladder for detecting bladder cancers [20, 21]. In essence, spiral CT, using single detector technology, was shown to be an excellent method for identifying virtually all anatomic abnormalities of the urinary tract with one exception: the upper tract urothelium. This one pitfall has been probably the single biggest reason for the continued use of IVU in patients with hematuria over the past decade. Prior to multi-detector technology, CT was limited in its ability to evaluate the urothelium because of limited spatial resolution relative to radiography, particularly in the coronal and sagittal planes. Nevertheless, the concept of CT urography has been introduced (prior to multi-detector technology) and refers to an exam that includes the CT evaluation of the renal paren-

Table 1. Brigham and Women's MSCT Urography Protocol

Phase range	Unenhanced abdominal/ pelvis	Nephrographic kidney	Urographic kidney-bladder
Tube voltage (kVp)	120	120	120
Tube current (mA)	330	500	330
Rotation time (s)	.5	.5	.5
Collimation (mm)	2.5	2.5	2.5
Section thickness (mm)	5	3	1.25
Increment (mm)	5	1.5	1
Display	Axial	Axial	Axial
			Coronal
			MIP

chyma and some method for visualizing the collecting system and ureter [22]. Some obtain CT following conventional IVU [23, 25], others obtain reformatted contrast material-enhanced coronal CT images [26, 27], and others obtain either a CT scout view or abdominal radiographs after a contrast-enhanced CT.

MSCT technology allows a CT urogram to be performed with CT alone. All of the technologic advantages cited above are exploited. Improved spatial resolution is used to better visualize the urothelium, improved speed and scan volume allow the entire urinary tract to be imaged with one acquisition, and increased flexibility allows data sets to be viewed in multiple ways.

We are currently investigating a novel protocol for MSCT urography (MSCTU, Table 1). We use it in patients with hematuria and suspected renal masses. All patients are administered water rather than iodinated contrast material orally. Three scan acquisitions are used. The first acquisition is obtained without intravenous contrast material and evaluates for urolithiasis. The second scan, obtained 100 s after IV contrast material and during the nephrographic phase, is performed mostly to detect and characterize renal masses. The third scan, obtained 8–10 min later, is performed to evaluate the collecting system and ureters (Fig. 1). Each scan is displayed in an axial format; the third scan is also displayed as coronal images. There are many possible protocols that could be used. Investigation is needed to determine the optimal protocol.

In addition to protocol optimization, there are several key issues that need to be addressed before MSCTU replaces IVU. The first issue is whether MSCTU can be used to visualize the intrarenal collecting system and ureters. This important feasibility step should determine whether the anatomy of the urinary tract and conventional IVU can be displayed. Second, test characteristics of MSCTU (e.g., sensitivity and specificity) need to be evaluated. Third, the issue of cost needs to be addressed to determine the impact of using CT rather than conventional IVU in patients with hematuria. Finally, since radiation exposure to patients during MSCTU is greater than during IVU, additional work needs to be done to determine the dose of various protocols and a consensus reached regarding whether the increased dose is justified. Techniques will need to be optimized to minimize radiation exposure to patients. This is an issue that concerns all of MSCT scanning.

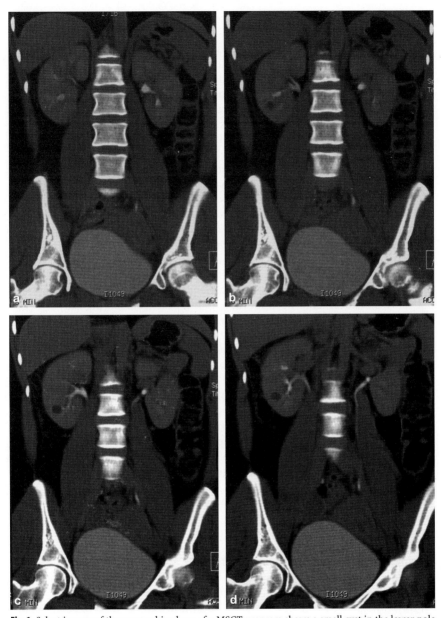

Fig. 1. Select images of the urographic phase of a MSCT urogram shows a small cyst in the lower pole of the right kidney

Renal Mass Evaluation

With the development of ultrasound and CT, cross-sectional imaging techniques became the standard way to confirm that a renal mass seen on IVU was benign. Work predominantly in the early 1980s demonstrated that conventional, non-spiral CT was the best test for detecting and characterizing renal masses [8, 9, 10]. With the advent of spiral CT, the entire kidney could be imaged without skip areas and improvements in small mass characterization were realized [15, 16]. However, our ability to detect all renal lesions seen at necropsy is still not possible. Although the detection of extremely small (i.e., $\leq$ 5 mm) lesions is limited, the rationale for doing so is somewhat suspect. Most of these lesions are benign. Furthermore, it has been shown that even if such small tumors are malignant, they are slow growing. Therefore, simply following them until they reach a sufficient size may be the most prudent approach [9]. In fact, finding additional small lesions that cannot be characterized may result in a cascade of unnecessary tests. There are two clinical scenarios for which increased detection of small renal masses may be of benefit. One is in patients with renal cell carcinoma for whom a partial nephrectomy is planned. Satellite foci of small renal carcinoma may exist in as many as 20% of nephrectomy specimens. Hence, identifying these additional sites of cancer may be important before nephron-sparing surgery [28]. Second, patients who are at increased risk for developing renal cell carcinoma (e.g., von Hippel-Lindau syndrome) may benefit by having their cancers detected earlier. Despite the theoretical advantages of spiral CT using single detector technology, to my knowledge, no studies have shown an increase in detection rate compared with conventional, non-spiral CT. Multi-detector technology may help in detecting more lesions using thinly collimated acquisitions. MSCT also has the possibility of improving the characterization of renal masses. Spiral CT has been shown to be of benefit in mass characterization, particularly in identifying small amounts of fat in suspected angiomyolipomas [16]. However, despite the advances in CT, approximately 5–10% of renal lesions remain indeterminate after full evaluation [29]. This results in non-diagnostic reports and subsequent follow-up CT scans and ultrasound examinations. The problem is further compounded by the fact that there is no known time interval by which we can be certain that a renal mass is benign. Therefore, if the characterization of small renal masses were improved, our reports would be more diagnostic and unnecessary and costly follow-up examinations avoided.

When imaging renal masses, a standard CT protocol utilizes 5-mm collimation. Because thinner collimation would improve spatial resolution and reduce partial volume averaging, protocols employing collimations less than 5 mm may improve the evaluation of small renal masses. MSCT can be used to obtain image data sets using 2.5-mm collimation of the entire kidney during a single breath hold. Whether viewing images with thinner slice thicknesses would improve the detection and characterization of renal masses awaits further evaluation.

Conclusion

While CT has emerged as the single most important imaging technique in the urinary tract, multi-detector technology is poised to increase the role of CT even further. Renal mass detection and characterization will likely be improved for patients with unexplained hematuria. MSCT presents sufficient technological advantages to allow the uroradiologist to consider eliminating the conventional intravenous urogram altogether and proceeding directly to CT. With further development of CT cystography, the MSCT urogram may ultimately serve as a single comprehensive evaluation of all anatomic abnormalities of the urinary tract.

References

1. Kalendar WA, Seissler W, Klotz E, Vock P (1990) Spiral volumetric CT with single-breath-hold technique, continuous transport, and continuous scanner rotation. Radiology 176:181–183
2. Klingenbeck-Regn K, Schaller S, Flohr T, Ohnesorge B, Kopp AF, Baum U (1999) Subsecond multi-slice computed tomography: basics and applications. Eur J Radiol 31:110–124
3. Sen S, Zincke H (1984) Value of excretory cystography in the diagnosis of bladder tumors. Br J Urol 56:499–501
4. Mushlin AI, Thornbury JR (1989) Intravenous pyelography: the case against its routine use. Ann Intern Med 111:58–70
5. Corwin HL, Silverstein MD (1988) The diagnosis of neoplasia in patients with asymptomatic hematuria: a decision analysis. J Urol 139:1002–1006
6. Lewis-Jones HG, Lamb GHR, Hughes PL (1989) Can ultrasound replace the intravenous urogram in preliminary investigation of renal tract disease? A prospective study. Br J Radiol 62:977–980
7. Warshauer DM, McCarthy SM, Street L, et al. (1988) Detection of renal masses: sensitivities and specificities of excretory urography/linear tomography, US and CT. Radiology 169:363–365
8. Amendola MA, Bree RL, Pollack HM et al. (1988) Small renal cell carcinomas: resolving a diagnostic dilemma. Radiology 166:637–741
9. Bosniak MA (1991) The small (≤ 3.0 cm) renal parenchymal tumor: detection, diagnosis, and controversies. Radiology 179:307–317
10. Dunnick NR. Renal lesions: great strides in imaging (1992) Radiology 182:305–306
11. Goldstein AS, Sclafani SJ, Kupferstein NH, Bass I, Lewis T, Panetta T, et al. (1985) The diagnostic superiority of computerized tomography. J Trauma 25:938–946
12. Cass AS, Viera J (1987) Comparison of IVP and CT findings in patients with suspected severe renal injury. Urology 29:484–487
13. Herschorn S, Radomski SB, Shoskes DA, Mahoney J, Hirshberg E, Klotz L (1991) Evaluation and treatment of blunt renal trauma. J Urol 146:274–276
14. Kawashima A, Sandler CM, Ernst RD, Goldman SM, Ravel B, Fishman EK (1997) Renal inflammatory disease: the current role of CT. Crit Rev Diagn Imaging 38:369–415
15. Silverman SG, Lee BY, Seltzer SE, Bloom DA, Corless CL, Adams, DF (1994) Small (≤ 3 cm) renal masses: correlation of spiral CT features and pathologic findings. AJR Am J Roentgenol 163:597–605
16. Silverman SG, Pearson GDN, Seltzer SE, Polger M, Tempany CMC, Adams DF, Brown DL, Judy PF (1996) Small (≤ 3 cm) hyperechoic renal masses: comparison of helical and conventional CT for diagnosing angiomyolipoma. AJR Am J Roentgenol 167:877–881
17. Smith RC, Rosenfield AT, Choe KA, et al. (1995) Acute flank pain: comparison of non-contrast enhanced CT and intravenous urography. Radiology 194:789–794
18. Rubin GD, Dake MD, Napel S, et al. (1994) Helical CT of renal artery stenosis: comparison of three-dimensional rendering techniques. Radiology 190:181–189
19. Figueroa K, Feurerstein D, Principe AL (1997) A comparison of three-dimensional spiral computed tomoangiography with renal angiography in the live-donor work-up. J Transpl Coord 7:195-198
20. Vining DJ; Zagoria RJ; Liu K, et al. (1996) CT cystoscopy: an innovation in bladder imaging. AJR Am J Roentgenol 166:409
21. Sommer FG, Olcott EW, Ch'en IY, Beaulieu CF (1997) Volume rendering of CT data: applications to the genitourinary tract. AJR Am J Roentgenol 168:1223–1226

22. Amis ES (z) Epitaph for the urogram. Radiology 213:639–640
23. Perlman ES, Rosenfield AT, Wexler JS, Glickman MG (1996) CT urography in the evaluation of urinary tract disease. J Comput Assist Tomogr 20:620–626
24. O'Malley ME, Toronto ON, Hahn PF, Yoder IC, McGovern FJ, Gazelle GS, Mueller PR (1999) Comparison of helical CT urography to IV urography for evaluation of patients with painless hematuria. Radiology 213 (P):474
25. Zawin ML, Egglin TK, Rosenfield AT (1999) Cost-effectiveness of CT urography in the evaluation of urinary tract abnormalities. Radiology 213 (P):474
26. Hoffman A, Ofer A, Nitecki S, et al (1997) Reconstructed CT ureteropyelography for accurate diagnosis of urinary tract lesions after kidney transplantation. Transplant Proc 29:2699–2700
27. McNicholas MM, Raptopoulos VD, Schwartz RDk, Sheiman RG, Zormpala A, et al. (1998) Excretory phase CT urography for opacification of the urinary collecting system. AJR Am J Roentgenol 170:1261–1267
28. Nissenkorn I, Bernheim J (1995) Multicentricity in renal cell carcinoma. J Urology 153:620–622
29. Kawashima A, Goldman SM, Sandler CM (1996) The indeterminate renal mass. Radiol Clin of North Am 34:997–1015

Application of Multislice Computed Tomography in Liver and Pancreas

Hoon Ji, Pablo R. Ros

Introduction

Multislice computed tomography (MSCT) allows us to obtain more rapid acquisition of images compared with spiral CT. With the combination of a multi-row detector ring and a fast gantry rotation time, the rate of section acquisition of MSCT can be up to 5–8 times faster than spiral CT [1]. In this chapter, we discuss the technical application of MSCT in the liver and pancreas and its impact in clinical protocols, including optimized scan parameters and enhancement strategies. In addition, with the rapid volume rendering of MSCT in conjunction with the development of three-dimensional (3D) software for viewing, a new era of CT-based abdominal visceral 3D imaging is becoming a reality.

Scanning Parameters

MSCT has an obvious impact on routine imaging protocols (collimation, pitch, and reconstruction interval), image quality (resolution and noise), use of intravenous contrast, filming, and other parameters. The most important key in all of these considerations is that the increased speed of imaging brings us closer to the dream of true isotropic volumetric imaging, with all of the advantages of tissue-specific volumetric rendering [2, 3].

Collimation

The practical considerations with regard to choice of collimation include spatial resolution, image noise, and length of coverage. The primary consideration should be the purpose of the study (i.e., appropriate for the structures being imaged). One can increase spatial resolution by decreasing the collimator width, but decreased collimator width also results in increased image noise and decreased length of coverage. Thus, several factors must be balanced to achieve the best result for a particular imaging problem. For example, the problem of limited length of coverage with decreased collimation width can be overcome by increasing pitch.

Pitch

In spiral CT, pitch is defined as the table feed distance per 360° rotation of the tube-detector apparatus divided by the collimator width. For MSCT, this definition can be extended to the table transport distance per rotation divided by the detector-row beam collimation. So, in the four multi-row detector CT, the spiral pitch 3.0 at 2.5-mm beam collimation will cover 7.5 mm per rotation. With MSCT, some pitches are preferred [4]. Selection of the pitches for MSCT is also affected by other conventional factors, such as the length of coverage versus the effective slice thickness and the ability to resolve small differences in tissue attenuation (contrast resolution).

For a given scan duration, minimizing collimation and maximizing pitch always results in the smallest effective slice thickness (i.e., highest spatial resolution). However, maximizing pitch also results in a decrease in contrast resolution. Thus, the most appropriate choice of scanning parameters depends upon the imaging problem under consideration. For example, because CT angiography (CTA) is an imaging study in which very high attenuation value-enhanced vascular structures are distinguished from the surrounding low attenuation value soft tissues (i.e., a high contrast resolution problem), the loss of contrast resolution caused by maximizing pitch (i.e., 6.0) can be disregarded. However, for CT of the liver, the potential loss of contrast resolution with maximal pitch must be taken into consideration. Liver and pancreas CT require both good spatial resolution and good contrast resolution. Therefore, a practical approach to liver and pancreas CT is to use relatively narrow collimation (such as 3–5 mm) and to increase pitch to 6.0 as needed to cover the entire liver.

Reconstruction Interval

Choice of reconstruction interval depends upon the clinical problem for which the study is being done. The smaller the reconstruction interval, the greater the longitudinal (z-axis) resolution. Therefore, if one is anticipating reconstructing multi-planar or 3D images from the spiral data set, a small reconstruction interval (with overlapping sections) is advantageous. However, if multi-planar or 3D images are not anticipated, contiguous (non-overlapping) reconstructions usually are adequate. Nevertheless, overlapping reconstructions have been shown to improve the detection of hepatic metastases and pulmonary nodules [5, 6, 7].

The practical tradeoff relates to maximizing longitudinal resolution versus limiting processing time, data storage, and the number of images to be reviewed (although these latter issues have become less problematic with improvements in computing speed and the use of µPACS workstations to view spiral CT data sets).

Contrast Media

Several studies have demonstrated that the volume of contrast medium used to enhance the thoracic vascular structures with spiral CT can be reduced by as much as one-half of that used for dynamic incremental CT [8, 9]. For abdominal CT, however, the issue of contrast medium reduction for spiral CT has not yet been resolved. This issue waits resolution, especially with MSCT because of its rapid scanning ability. However, the most important patient-related factor affecting the magnitude of hepatic contrast enhancement is body weight [10]. Oral contrast is used, same as for conventional spiral CT, but in cases in which hypervascular tumors are suspected or when considering CTA, water is recommended as an oral contrast agent.

Enhancement Strategies

Scan Timing

The appropriate scan delay for spiral CT depends on the contrast medium injection protocol used. The timing of peak aortic and hepatic contrast enhancement depends primarily on the injection duration [11, 12]. Rapid or low-volume (shorter duration) injections produce earlier peak enhancement, whereas slow- or high-volume (longer duration) injections result in later peak enhancement. Thus, if a fixed scan delay is used, these factors must be taken into account.

In our practice, a preliminary mini bolus (5 ml/sec for 4 s) with one scan every 2 s beginning 10 s after the beginning of injection can be used. Time to aortic peak is determined from the resultant time attenuation curve and is used as the injection to scan delay for multi-phase imaging. However, the scan delay can be timed more accurately with a bolus tracking software program [13].

Liver

MSCT may demonstrate three distinct hepatic circulatory phases with the triple pass technique (Fig. 1) [14, 15]. The first imaging pass provides a true (or early) arterial phase and enhancement of hypervascular neoplasms. The second pass corresponds in timing to initial opacification of the portal venous system and is labeled a "parenchymal (or late arterial) phase". The enhancement of hypervascular neoplasms is maximized during this imaging pass. For both primary and metastatic hypervascular neoplasms, such as hepatocellular carcinoma, islet cell tumor, carcinoid, and sarcoma, approximately 30% more lesions are detectable on the arterial dominant phase than on the delayed phase of enhancement [16, 17, 18, 19].

In the third imaging pass, hepatic veins that have been unenhanced in both the early arterial phase and parenchymal phase are enhanced. In addition, enhancement of background hepatic parenchyma is maximized. Acquisition timing corresponds to what has been conventionally labeled as the "portal venous phase". Since this corresponds in timing to conventional hepatic CT scanning, it has been termed the "hepatic venous phase". Tumors that are hyperattenuating on the arterial phase and parenchymal phase may become isoattenuating or hypoattenuating on the hepatic venous phase [15, 16, 17]. In

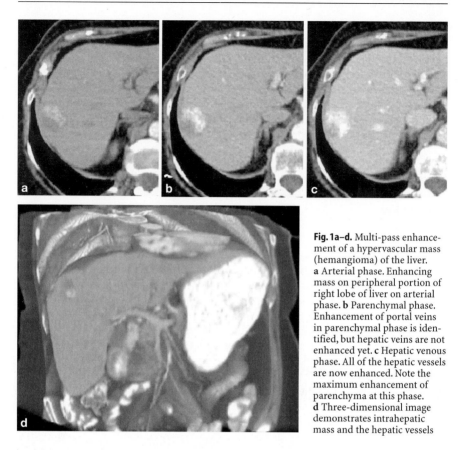

Fig. 1a–d. Multi-pass enhancement of a hypervascular mass (hemangioma) of the liver. **a** Arterial phase. Enhancing mass on peripheral portion of right lobe of liver on arterial phase. **b** Parenchymal phase. Enhancement of portal veins in parenchymal phase is identified, but hepatic veins are not enhanced yet. **c** Hepatic venous phase. All of the hepatic vessels are now enhanced. Note the maximum enhancement of parenchyma at this phase. **d** Three-dimensional image demonstrates intrahepatic mass and the hepatic vessels

patients having surveillance studies following surgery, ablative therapy, or chemoembolization, in which CT arteriography is not necessary, only the second and third imaging passes are used.

Pancreas

For pancreatic imaging, biphasic techniques, such as spiral CT, are usually used with an arterial phase at a 40-s delay and a venous phase at a 70-s delay time after a 100 ml volume of contrast has been injected at 3 ml/s (Table 1). In the evaluation of patients with a suspected pancreatic mass, multi-phasic enhancement is used with initial arterial and parenchymal phase obtained at a 20-s and a 40-s delay time, respectively, after a 100 ml volume of contrast has been injected at 4 ml/sec. A hepatic venous phase is then obtained at 70 s. The arterial and parenchymal phases are limited to coverage of the porta-hepatic and pancreas. The hepatic venous phase covers the entire abdomen, including the liver (Fig. 2).

Mean differences of enhancement between tumor and normal pancreas are greater in the optimal pancreatic phase than in the hepatic venous phase. Enhan-

Table 1. A MSCT protocol for the liver and pancreas

Protocol	Indications	po	IV rate/ vol.	Delay (s)	Area	Collimation (mm)	Feed (mm)	Reconstruction (thk /int)	Remarks
Liver									
Basic liver	Suspect liver mets	C+	3/100	35 60	Liver A/P	2.5	15	5/5	For gastric cancer, po citrocarbinate
Hypervascular liver lesion	Hypervascular metastasis search (HCC, FNH, hemangioma, etc.)	H₂O	4/100	20/25 60	Liver A/P	2.5	15	5/3	
Pancreas									
Basic pancreas	Pancreatitis, suspect pancreatic necrosis	C+	3/100	40 70	Pancreas A/P	2.5	15	5/5 3/1.5	
Pancreatic mass	Suspect pancreatic mass: jaundice	H₂O	4/100	20/40 70	Pancreas A/P	1 2.5	6 6	1.25/1 3/2.5	

C+, 2.1% dilution of barium sulfate; H_2O, water; IV, intravenous; A/P, abdomen to pelvis; thk, thickness; int, interval; HCC, hepatocellular carcinoma; FNH, focal nodular hyperplasia

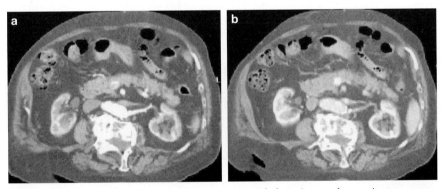

Fig. 2a, b. Biphasic enhancement of normal pancreas. Curved planar images show entire pancreas on the pancreatic (a) and portal phase (b) of enhancement. Note the good visibility of the peripancreatic vessels

cement of the critical vascular structures in the pancreatic phase is also useful in staging and predicting which patients will have surgically unresectable tumors [20, 21, 22].

The other areas of the greatest clinical impact of MSCT have been the evaluation of trauma patients and the expanded anatomic coverage during CTA. This facilitates the diagnosis of vascular disease or active arterial extravasation by scanning during peak contrast opacification. The extent to which these novel applications will play a role in the day-to-day evaluation of patients with liver and pancreas disease awaits the results of scientific inquiry.

Sample Protocol with Four Multi-Row Detector CT

Liver

In our practice, bolus injection for multi-pass imaging is 4 ml/s for 25 s of 60% nonionic contrast material (30 g iodine). Two passes during the arterial phase can be obtained: true arterial phase (10 s after contrast arrives in the abdominal aorta) and parenchymal arterial phase (30–40 s after the initiation of contrast).

Table speed for the single breath hold first and second pass back-to-back acquisitions is 15 mm/s. Image thickness is 3 mm for the first pass and 3 mm or 5 mm for the second pass. A third imaging pass, beginning 60 s after the beginning of injection and employing a table speed of 15 mm/s corresponds in timing with the conventional "portal venous phase" to evaluate the remainder of the abdomen (Table 1).

Pancreas

For pancreatic evaluation, we prefer to use 600 ml water as an oral contrast 30 min prior to scanning. Two passes of the enhancement are usually taken. The first pass is taken with 1.25-mm thickness on a 35-s delay after 3 ml/s for 33 s injection of 60% iodinated contrast. The second pass, portal venous phase scan, used to be taken 70 s after contrast injection with 2.5-mm scan thickness. The CT data is then transferred to a workstation, where image reformatting is done (Fig. 3).

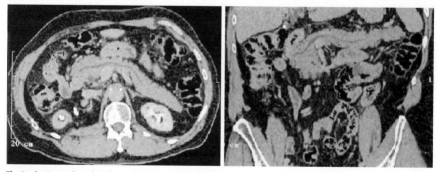

Fig. 3a, b. Curved multi-planar images along the pancreatic duct (a and b). Note the mild dilatation of the pancreatic duct

3D Imaging

With the rapid scanning ability of MSCT, it is feasible to obtain a 3D data set of the entire liver during a single breath hold, analogous to a 3D magnetic resonance (MR) data set. By reconstructing these data on a work station, excellent quality 3D images may be obtained (Fig. 3 and Fig. 4). We have found the image

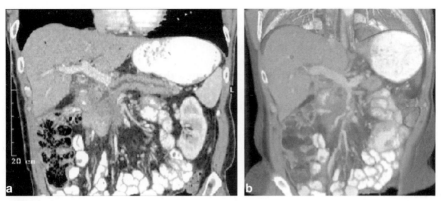

Fig. 4a, b. Ductal adenocarcinoma of pancreas. **a** Ill-defined mass in the head of the pancreas with dilatation of duct is demonstrated on the curved planar image along the pancreatic duct. **b** Three-dimensional image shows encasement of the superior mesenteric vein

quality in the reconstructed sagittal, coronal, or curved planes to be excellent in most cases. Curved multi-planar imaging along the dilated biliary tree or vessels may more clearly elucidate the anatomy and pathology than axial imaging alone.

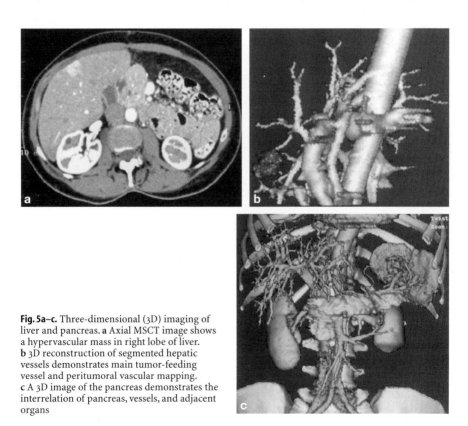

Fig. 5a–c. Three-dimensional (3D) imaging of liver and pancreas. **a** Axial MSCT image shows a hypervascular mass in right lobe of liver. **b** 3D reconstruction of segmented hepatic vessels demonstrates main tumor-feeding vessel and peritumoral vascular mapping. **c** A 3D image of the pancreas demonstrates the interrelation of pancreas, vessels, and adjacent organs

Such unique imaging of the liver and pancreas may improve lesion detection, characterization, and surgical planning (Fig. 5) [4]. For example, curved planar images along the pancreatic duct may nicely clarify the relationship of tumors to the pancreatic parenchyma and duct. Ductal abnormalities can be nicely delineated (Fig. 4). Such curved planar imaging along the pancreatic duct has proven useful in evaluating the patient prior to the Puestow procedure [23]. In addition, MSCT may perform dynamic subtraction CT of the liver during a single breath hold, which may be an elegant means to quantify vascularity. Such enhancement may be a reflection of the biological activity of a tumor [24].

Limitations of MSCT

The net result of MSCT is that many more thinly collimated scans are routinely obtained. For certain types of examinations, such as CTA, the image files are extraordinarily large with up to 1000 slices. It becomes impractical to view these large data sets on film. Tracking through the images at a PACS station is the most efficient way to review the large amount of data obtained with MSCT. Although cone beam artifacts are theoretically a potential problem of MSCT, they have not caused significant image degradation to date.

Timing of the scan acquisition becomes more critical as the increased speed of MSCT narrows the "temporal window" for desirable phase of enhancement. Without proper timing for abdominal studies, it is possible to scan too early and miss the peak portal venous. These different circulatory phases can only be separated by precisely timing the start of acquisition with the individual patient circulation time.

References

1. Berland LL, Smith JK (1998) Multidetector array CT: once again technology creates new opportunities. Radiology 209:327–329
2. Hu H, He HD, Foley WD, Fox SH (2000) Four multidetector-row helical CT: image quality and volume coverage speed. Radiology 215:55–62
3. Wong K, Nelson RC, Hinton ST, et al. (1999) Single breath-hold high-resolution three-dimensional CT of the liver using multidetector helical technology. Radiology 213 (P):125
4. Hu H (1999) Multislice helical CT: scan and reconstruction. Med Physics 26:5–18
5. Weg N, Scheer MR, Gabor MP (1998) Liver lesions: improved detection with dual detector array CT and routine 2.5 mm thin collimation. Radiology 209:417–426
6. Buckley JA, Scott WWJ, Siegelman SS, et al. (1995) Pulmonary nodules: effect of increased data sampling on detection with spiral CT and confidence in diagnosis. Radiology 196:395–400
7. Urban BA, Fishman EK, Kuhlman JE, Kawashima A, Hennessey JG, Siegelman SS (1993) Detection of focal hepatic lesions with spiral CT: comparison of 4- and 8-mm interscan spacing. AJR Am J Roentgenol 160:783–785
8. Costello P, Dupuy ED, Ecker CP, Tello R (1992) Spiral CT of the thorax with reduced volume of contrast material: a comparative study. Radiology 183:663–666
9. Costello P, Ecker CP, Tello R, Hartnell GG (1992) Assessment of the thoracic aorta by spiral CT. AJR Am J Roentgenol 158:1127–1130
10. Heiken JP, Brink JA, McClennan BL, Sagel SS, Crowe TM, Gaines MV (1995) Dynamic incremental CT: effect of volume and concentration of contrast material and patient weight on hepatic enhancement. Radiology 195:353–357
11. Heiken JP, Brink JA, McClennan BL, Sagel SS, Forman HP, DiCroce J (1993) Dynamic contrast-enhanced CT of the liver: comparison of contrast medium injection rates and uniphasic and biphasic injection protocols. Radiology 187:327–331

12. Chambers TP, Baron RL, Lush RM (1994) Hepatic CT enhancement. II. Alterations in contrast material volume and rate of injection within the same patients. Radiology 193:518–523
13. Silverman PM, Roberts SC, Ducic I, et al. (1996) Assessment of a technology that permits individualized scan delays on helical hepatic CT: a technique to improve efficiency in use of contrast material. AJR Am J Roentgenol 167:79–84
14. Mitsuzaki K, Yamashita Y, Ogata I, Nishiharu T, Urata J, Takahashi M (1996) Multiphase helical CT of the liver for detecting small hepatomas in patients with liver cirrhosis: contrast injection protocol and optimal timing. AJR Am J Roentgenol 167:753–757
15. Paulson EK, McDermott VG, Keogan MT, DeLong DM, Frederick MG, Nelson RC (1998) Carcinoid metastases to the liver: role of triple phase helical CT. Radiology 206:143–150
16. Larson RE, Semelka RC, Bagley AS, Molina PL, Brown ED, Lee JKT (1994) Hypervascular malignant liver lesions: comparison of various MR imaging pulse sequences and dynamic CT. Radiology 192:393–399
17. Kopka L, Rodenwaldt I, Fischer U, Mueller DW, Oestmann W, Grabbe E (1996) Dual phase helical CT of the liver: effects of bolus tracking and different volumes of contrast material. Radiology 201:321–326
18. Oliver IH, Baron RL, Federle MP, Jones BC, Sheng R (1997) Hypervascular liver metastases: do unenhanced and hepatic arterial phase CT images effect tumor detection. Radiology 205:709–715
19. Baron RL, Oliver IH, Dodd GD, Nalesnik M, Holbert BL, Carr B (1996) Hepatocellular carcinoma: evaluation with biphasic contrast enhanced helical CT. Radiology 199:505–511
20. Boland GW, O'Malley ME, Saez M, Fernandez-del-Castillo C, Warshaw AL, Mueller PR (1999) Pancreatic-phase versus portal vein-phase helical CT of the pancreas: optimal temporal window for evaluation of pancreatic adenocarcinoma. AJR Am J Roentgenol 172:605–608
21. O'Malley ME, Boland GW, Wood BJ, Fernandez-del-Castillo C, Warshaw AL, Mueller PR (1999) Adenocarcinoma of the head of the pancreas: determination of surgical unresectability with thin-section pancreatic-phase hellical CT. AJR Am J Roentgenol 173:1513–1518
22. Tabuchi T, Itoh K, Ohshio G, Kojima N, Maetani Y, Shibata T, Konishi J (1999) Tumor staging of pancreatic adenocarcinoma using early- and late-phase helical CT. AJR Am J Roentgenol 173:375–380
23. Raptopoulos V, Prassopoulos P, Chuttani R, et al. (1998) Multiplanar CT pancreatography in distal cholangiography with minimum intensity projections. Radiology 207:317–324
24. Nelson RC, Johnson GA, Spielman AL, et al. (1999) Single breath-hold dynamic subtraction CT of the liver using multidetector helical technology. Radiology 213:125

Virtual Endoscopy

Didier Bielen, Dirk Vanbeckevoort, Maarten Thomeer, Marc Peeters

Introduction

Although endoscopy has existed for a long time, it is the nearly exclusive domain of the endoscopist, a doctor trained in internal medicine. Using video-assisted technology, endoscopy is used to view the inner surface of hollow organs in a continuous fashion (mostly colon, stomach or the tracheobronchial tree). Because endoscopy yields detailed anatomical information of the inner surface of a displayed wall segment, the technique is ideal for detecting mucosal lesions [1, 2]. In 1994, Vining first described the virtual colonography [2]. The radiologist, however, became interested in visualising the inner surface of liquid filled spaces (e.g. the bladder), vascular structures and even the intracranial cisterns in a three-dimensional (3D) manner, rather than just visualising air-filled hollow organs.

Classic 3D imaging presents an object as if one were holding it in one's hand [3]. Unlike the adjective, 'virtual' could suggest a non-existing world – a computer generated reality. The virtual endoscopic technique offers a fly-through method, as if one were in an endoscope, thereby combining the features of endoscopy and cross-sectional volumetric imaging that has been generated using either computed tomography (CT) or magnetic resonance imaging [4].

This chapter will discuss the general principles of image acquisition using CT and different 3D image display techniques. Clinical application domains in gastroenterology, where virtual endoscopy actually is or can be used, will be illustrated.

General Principles of Data Acquisition

The ultimate method for performing virtual endoscopy is not yet determined. Many variations in the performance of 3D rendering exist [5].

However, all routine CT imaging techniques that provide high-resolution cross-sectional images can be post-processed to obtain 3D reconstructions [1]. Continuously rotating spiral CT systems are now a day best suited, be it a single or multi-slice detector system.

Proposed technique parameters, as mentioned in the literature, are listed in Table 1. Optimal 3D image rendering requires high-resolution data acquisition, in-plane (x- and y-axis) and through-plane (z-axis): voxels should be (nearly)

Table 1. Acquisition parameters for three dimensional image rendering

Organ	Technique	Collimation	Rotation	Pitch	mA (s)	Reconstruction	Author
Colon	SCT	3 mm	NA	1.5	NA	2 mm	Laghi et al. [9]
Colon	MSCT	Four 1-mm thick slices	0.5 s	6	150 mAs	2 mm	Laghi et al. [10]
Colon	MSCT	Four 2.5-mm thick slices	0.75 s	8	20–70 mAs	1 mm	Thomeer/ Vanbeckevoort (KULeuven)
Colon	MSCT	5 mm	0.8 s	3	50 mA	3 mm	Fletcher and Luboldt (Mayo Clinic) [22]
Colon	MSCT	1 mm	0.5 s	6	120 mAs	0.8 mm	Fletcher and Luboldt (University of Tübingen) [22]
Stomach	SCT	3 mm	0.75 s	1.5	223 mA	1–1.5 mm	Lee [29]
Stomach	SCT	3 mm	1 s	1.3–2	180–220 mAs	1 mm	Ogata et al. [8]

CT, computed tomography; SCT, Single-slice CT; MSCT, multislice CT; NA, not available

isotropic, i.e. having the same dimensions and resolution in the three directions and being as small as possible. Using spiral CT, however, the effective slice thickness (EST) is greater than the collimation width, and this is proportional to pitch, thereby reducing the longitudinal spatial resolution in the z-axis.

The longitudinal resolution is considered adequate when the EST is less than or equal to the lesion diameter [6]. This longitudinal resolution can be maximised, however, with images that are reconstructed with overlap. For imaging applications that require maximal longitudinal resolution, single-detector spiral CT images should be reconstructed with at least 60% overlap relative to the effective slice thickness [7]. Use of highly overlapping source images (87–90%) is not necessary to generate 3D images [8].

Optimal section spacing for multislice CT (MSCT) systems needs to be established [7]. With MSCT, however, either the scan time can be reduced dramatically compared with conventional spiral CT, with consequent dose reduction [9, 10], or the volume to be investigated can be extended. The volume coverage speed of a four MSCT can be at least twice as fast with fully comparable image quality or, in many cases, three times as fast with diagnostically comparable image quality [11].

Different Techniques of Imaging Display

Virtual endoscopy, a type of interactive 3D medical imaging, allows physicians to navigate through computer simulations of the human body, based on volumetric data acquisition. The ultimate method for performing and displaying virtual endoscopy is yet to be determined. Many authors proposed different imaging techniques, mostly concerning colonic imaging. One of the most cumbersome challenges that await investigators is how accurate and reproducible rendering techniques are in the demonstration of normal and abnormal anatomy.

3D renderings could not have been developed without the advances in computer hardware, software and display technologies. 3D imaging offers an integration of the axial CT sections in a form that is easier to interpret than the original images. The volume of data is represented in a 2D plane with respect to spatial relationship by means of visual cues. Each of these rendering techniques is based on complex mathematical models. Projecting lines (rays) through the 3D data sets, thereby analysing the voxels they are passing, generates these 2D representations. Differences in rendering techniques depend on the manner in which voxels are selected and weighted [12].

Of the different 3D imaging techniques currently available for virtual endoscopy, we describe the principles, advantages and disadvantages. Comparison of different imaging facilities, as studied by some authors, should help the radiologist to choose the most adapted modality, given available computer facilities, time needed for computational work and review time.

Shaded-Surface Display

The complex process of shaded-surface display (SSD), mostly performed on dedicated workstations, consists of several steps [1, 13]. Many manufacturers have developed their own hardware and software for these tasks.

The first step toward surface rendering is segmentation i.e. isolating the organ of interest from the surroundings. The chief requirement to obtain an adequate endoscopic view is sufficient image contrast between the voxels to be viewed and those comprising the viewpoint. SSDs therefore rely on the thresholding of the data to create a model in which a binary classification is made either keeping or deleting voxels from the data set. A voxel is classified on the basis of the signal intensity of the original data. That threshold must be carefully chosen, based on the signal intensity in the anatomy of interest. For example, CT voxels with a Hounsfield number equal to 200 are considered to be bone, whereas those with a Hounsfield number less than –400 are considered to be air (Fig. 1). Using interactive erosion or dilation, the tissue or organ of interest is further isolated from the surroundings.

Once the voxels in the image data are labelled, a mathematical model of the surface is extracted. For any given view direction, an image is created that shades or colours the surface in proportion to the amount of light it would reflect from a simulated light source back to the observer and may darken the reflections in proportion to distance.

The advantages of surface rendering include superior speed and flexibility, because the size of the data set is greatly reduced when creating a surface model; hardware and software requirements are less demanding. One of the major disadvantages, however, is that reducing the volume data to isodense surfaces eliminates the wide range of density values inherent in the CT data. Such displays cannot simultaneously represent voxels with a range of attenuation values. Surfaces are created with only a small percentage of the available data, which is a common

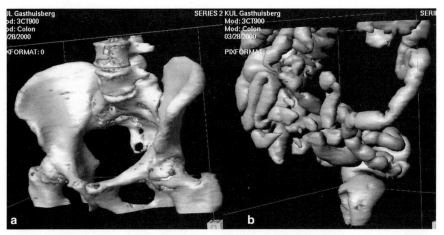

Fig. 1a, b. Influence of thresholding in shaded-surface display. **a** Thresholding set to bone (200 HU). **b** Thresholding set to air (–400 HU)

criticism of the technique. In addition, surface rendering is not adequate for the visualisation of structures that do not have naturally well-differentiated surfaces (e.g. air vs bowel wall) [12].

Volume Rendering

Similar to the other techniques, the volume-rendering (VR) technique builds up a 3D image by casting mathematical rays in some desired viewing direction through a stack of reconstructed slices. These renderings can be done using either parallel or divergent rays.

Parallel ray casting is mathematically equivalent to locating the observer at an infinite distance from the observed object. Using divergent rays, nonparallel rays radiating from the observer's location, perspective is added to the volume, lending objects the impression of relative positions, shape and distance [14].

The VR technique takes the entire volume of the data, sums the contribution of each voxel along the ray and displays the resulting value for each pixel of the display. As a first step, the volume may be segmented by eliminating surrounding structures that are not of interest. Reducing the effective size of the data set helps to accelerate the process of rendering.

VR typically segments the data set on the basis of voxel attenuation values represented by a density histogram. Adjusting window width and level, as commonly used in displaying axial images, displays soft tissues, bones and lungs. A change in width alters the contrast, whereas a change in level alters the data inclusion and the attenuation of voxels in the resulting image. A transfer function converts the attenuation values, i.e. Hounsfield units, to lighting properties, such as opacity, brightness and colour.

Opacity is a measure of the degree in which structures that appear closer to the observer obscure structures that seem farther away. A low opacity value

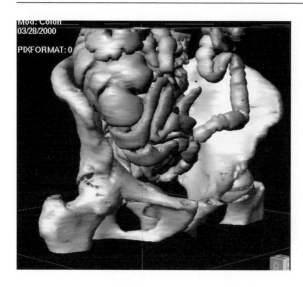

Fig. 2. Volume rendering showing both pelvis (bone) and the colon (air) simultaneously

allows the user to see through structures, because they seem to be transparent. A high opacity value produces images with an appearance like that of a SSD. Varying the opacity also affects the apparent object size. Higher opacity values make objects look larger, whereas lower opacity makes them look smaller. Brightness settings affect the appearance of the image. However, they are subjective and depend on the preferences of the individual user.

Colour is assigned to simulate expected normal tissue colour in vivo, based on the assumption that voxels representing a given tissue have a characteristic attenuation value with a Gaussian distribution of intensities around a central peak value. Each distribution is approximated by means of a trapezoid in the software. Multiple trapezoidal distributions can be displayed simultaneously, thereby displaying different objects of interest (Fig. 2). These manipulations can be performed in real time, which allows for the making of minor adjustments in the parameters without waiting for lengthy processing. Other display techniques, however, are possible.

Computer technologies can generate a fly-through image, placing the observers' viewpoint inside the organ of interest. For gastrointestinal structures, this creates the endoscopy-like images [15]. Navigation within the volume is accomplished by creating a so-called flight pad, the line on which the virtual camera moves. This flight pad can be generated either manually, or it can be computer assisted [15, 16, 17]. VR images of the camera's view are created along the flight pad, using a certain field of view (FOV) and a camera direction. In the classical endoscopic view, the camera, with a FOV of, for example, 60° is directed along the axis of the investigated structure. When oriented perpendicular to the wall of the structure, the so-called panoramic view [16] is generated.

Other visualisation methods, however, can be used, e.g. cylindrical and planar map projections, as mentioned in the literature [18]. A movie can be composed using the consecutive camera views along the flight pad in a forward and/or reverse order.

Ray Sum Display

As in SSD, all pixels other than specific threshold values (e.g. –400 HU) are removed automatically. Contiguous pixels at the boundary are modelled as a surface. In SSD, only the first voxel encountered along the imaginary projection ray that is above the user-defined threshold is selected as the inner surface of the investigated organ. In the ray sum projection, however, the sum of the pixels of the threshold range is modelled, resulting in a membrane-like appearance similar to that seen in conventional double-contrast barium examinations. This allows abnormalities of the bowel wall to be seen through the surface and the other overlying structures [8].

Tissue Transition Projection

The tissue transition projection (TTP) is an imaging process that visualises only the differences in attenuation values of neighbouring voxels concerning the voxels in the whole volume, similar to VR. These differences in density must be high enough to allow segmentation of the lumen. It is irrelevant whether or not the lumen shows a negative or positive contrast to the surroundings. The TTP enhances surface transitions while suppressing homogeneous areas; through transparent display, a delineation of bowel wall similar to conventional double-contrast studies is realised (Fig. 3) [19]. This technique bares the advantage of presenting the entire bowel, hence supporting the anatomical orientation. The sensitivity for detection of mucosal detail remains to be determined [20].

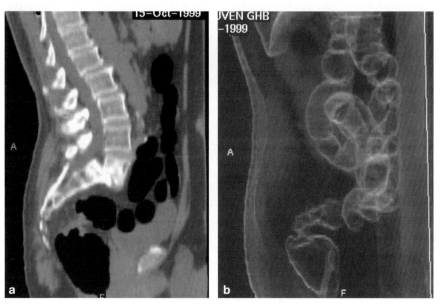

Fig. 3a, b. Computed tomography colonography using multi-planar reformation (a) and tissue transition projection (b)

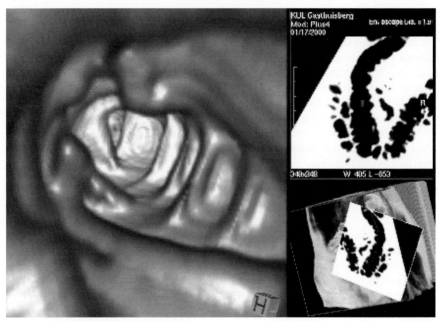

Fig. 4. Multi display virtual colonoscopy

Comparison of Different Techniques

As studied by Hopper et al. [21], virtual reality is best with VR when compared with SSD, because it provides better mucosal detail. Additionally, with VR, the entire spiral CT volume is used, which allows voxels to be grouped into multiple categories on the basis of their attenuation values (using multiple trapezoids) and these groups to be reconstructed as separate structures. The TTP displays a delineation of bowel wall similar to conventional double-contrast studies [19]. This technique bares the advantage of presenting the entire bowel, hence supporting the anatomical orientation.

Optimal software should provide real-time interactivity. A split screen displays virtual endoscopic viewing and correlated 2D images in a multi-format window (Fig. 4). The 2D images can be either the native axial images stacked together to create the volume at the time of acquisition or multi-planar reconstructions, i.e. cuts along orthogonal planes. The combined approach of 2D and 3D endoscopic views improves the diagnostic performance [9, 22].

Clinical Applications

Virtual Colonoscopy

Virtual colonoscopy is a relatively new method for visualisation of the colon based on the above-mentioned post-processing of MSCT 3D volumetric acquired data. The coupling of rapid data acquisition and advanced 3D rendering techniques has led to the introduction of virtual colonoscopy as a possible screening tool for colorectal cancer, knowing that colorectal cancer is a medium term evolution of benign polyps.

To prove effective in reducing mortality, the screening method should demonstrate a high diagnostic accuracy at a low cost and prove to be safe and highly acceptable to patients. Virtual colonoscopy promises to be a safe, fast and a relatively low-invasive method for detecting polyps and other tumorous lesions [22]. The patient has to be prepared with a routine bowel preparation, e.g. Prepacol (Codali, Belgium) before the CT scan to cleanse the bowel of residual stool and liquid. This preparation seems to be the most important barrier to patient compliance.

A spiral acquisition is performed in a single breath hold after retrograde inflation of air or carbon dioxide; the latter improves compliance through the faster absorption rate. The so-created important difference in contrast between the colon wall and the lumen makes this interface an easy target for the different rendering techniques. Furthermore, MSCT has just been introduced and will reduce the examination time.

Different bowel relaxants, e.g. glucagon (Glucagen Novo Nordisk Pharma, Belgium) or butyl hyoscine (Buscopan Boehringer Ingelheim, Belgium), have been administered intravenously to allow for better distension and to reduce the colonic spasm. However, disagreement still exists in the literature.

A localising scanogram is performed to assess colonic distension. If necessary, additional air is administered, and the scanogram is repeated until adequate distension is achieved. Different acquisition parameters are proposed in the literature (Table 1). For maximising mucosal detail and to proceed with a realistic detailed view of polyps, a narrow beam collimation is the most crucial factor. Collimation thickness of 3–5 mm and a pitch of 1.3–2.0 are currently used. Depending on the chosen parameters, certain artefacts can show up less or more (smoothing artefacts, stair step artefacts, longitudinal blurring and distortion). Although a pitch of 2.0 causes some blurring and distortion, no major differences are seen with a pitch of 1.0.

The use of both the supine and prone positions for patients undergoing CT colonography decreases the number of collapsed segments, hence improving evaluation of the colon and increases the sensitivity for polyp detection [23]. An alternative is to tag the residual stool and liquid by means of a previously orally administered contrast agent. Electronic cleansing of the bowel, so-called subtraction CT colonoscopy, is under investigation [24]. This could make the patient's preparation unnecessary.

The use of iodinated contrast agents for faecal tagging, however, is still contested. Prone scanning may obviate the need for oral contrast by eliminating errors due to excess colonic fluid or residual stool. Dose reduction is of primary importance, moreover, if virtual colonoscopy would be used as a possible screening tool.

The use of an effective tube current of 100 mA or less in order to become an acceptable radiation exposure is advised. There is no significant decrease in polyp detection when lowering the tube current to 70 mA [25]. In our experience, a dose even as low as 20 mA does not compromise image interpretation. At

70 mA, the radiation dose for CT performed in both supine and prone positions is similar to the dose for a barium enema. The strategy used to view the data set can vary. Most radiologists perform retro- and antegrade fly-throughs and correlate 3D endoluminal findings with reformatted images. Subsequently, the colon is re-examined by scrolling through each of the three orthogonal reformats following the course of the large bowel.

Clinical studies have examined CT colonography as a potential screening tool for colorectal neoplasm and as a method for evaluating patients with an incomplete colonoscopy. Preliminary results indicate that the accuracy of virtual colonoscopy exceeds that of the barium enema and approximates that of conventional colonoscopy. The sensitivity for detecting patients with polyps greater than 10 mm is 85% or greater in all of the studies, with a corresponding specificity almost always greater than 90%. The sensitivity for detecting polyps equal to 10 mm was 75% or greater in every study [22]. In 100 patients, Fenlon et al. found a sensitivity of 91% for polyps that were 10 mm or more, 82% of the polyps between 6 mm and 9 mm and 55% for polyps that were 5 mm or smaller [26].

An important question is whether the low rate of sensitivity for the detection of lesions smaller than 10 mm is acceptable. There is still controversy if polyps smaller than 10 mm are of clinical importance. Moreover, the probability of cancer is low in this subgroup.

Although these findings suggest that virtual colonoscopy has a lower sensitivity than conventional colonoscopy, one must keep in mind that 10–20% of the colonic polyps may be missed using conventional colonoscopy. Lesions hidden by haustral folds can be discerned using virtual colonoscopy due to the specific ability of retrograde viewing. In the case of colonic cancer, virtual endoscopy is able to detect additional lesions, especially when conventional colonoscopy can not pass an obstructing tumour.

The ability to perform polypectomy and the higher accuracy attributed to colonoscopy are advantages which favour colonoscopy over colonography for screening. Thus, if colonography is to become a routine screening method, then increasing the accuracy in colonography by improving data acquisition and analysis is of great importance.

Virtual Gastroscopy

Virtual endoscopic techniques using volumetric spiral CT can evaluate gastric tumours and other abnormalities. Possible indications are early or advanced gastric cancer and lymphoma (Fig. 5) and submucosal tumours, such as leiomyoma [22]. The required contrast difference between the gastric wall and its lumen can be enhanced by ingestion of effervescent granules containing tartaric acid (e.g. Zoru, E-Z-Em, Belgium). Maximal gastric distension is achieved by administering a bowel relaxant (e.g. glucagon (Glucagen Novo Nordisk Pharma, Belgium) or tiemonium iodide (Visceralgine Forte Exel Pharma, Belgium).

Using diluted contrast or double contrast technique, virtual CT gastroscopy showed artefacts; these can mimic polyps, erosions or flat ulcers [27]. Although benefiting the non-invasiveness of the technique, a few limitations have been

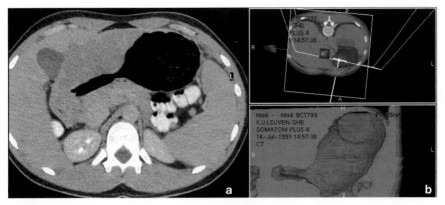

Fig. 5a, b. Virtual gastroscopy showing lymphoma. **a** Axial image and **b** shaded-surface display

reported. Flat or small lesions are difficult to detect. Gastric residual fluid or food can hinder endoscopic analysis and can be confused with pathologic changes. The inability to obtain samples is a further obstacle. The capability of performing simultaneous evaluation of mucosal changes and extraluminal abnormalities is, however, a unique feature of this technique.

Small Bowel

The small bowel has traditionally been a difficult area to evaluate. Even for endoscopy, it remains a challenge despite advances in fibre-optic techniques: a major part remains inaccessible. Small bowel enema currently represents the only reliable technique. Even for adequate CT evaluation and for performing virtual endoscopy of the small bowel, complete filling of the entire bowel is mandatory. This requires the use of a duodenal tube followed by the application of oral radiodense contrast mixed with methylcellulose [28].

The high contrast between the bowel content and the wall permits VR and endoscopic imaging, although navigation still challenges the virtual endoscopist. Pathologic changes in inflammatory bowel disease, such as thickened folds or cobblestone in Crohn's disease, are better seen from the inside.

Conclusion

Based on a volume data set, acquired using MSCT, 3D rendering allows a realistic display of many anatomical and pathological structures. Using SSD or VR, intra-abdominal structures, such as the colon, stomach and small bowel, can be imaged in a perspective or endoscopic way.

Most investigations, until today, concern colonic imaging. Virtual colonoscopy promises to be a valuable technique in screening non-symptomatic persons for colonic polyps, as compared with the classical colonoscopy, today's gold standard. Further improvements are, however, required concerning patient preparation, sensitivity and specificity and image processing. As first and most extensively investigated in the colon, applying comparable virtual endoscopic techniques for the stomach and small bowel opens new perspectives in a non-invasive imaging of these organs.

Acknowledgements. Special thanks to Sven Bollue for image data processing and creating the 3D models on a Silicon Graphics Workstation (Silicon Graphics, Mountain View, Calif.) with Siemens 3DVirtuoso Software (Siemens, Erlangen, Germany).

References

1. Jolesz FA, Lorensen WE et al. (1997) Interactive virtual endoscopy. AJR Am J Roentgenol 169:1229–1235
2. Vining DJ, Winston-Salem NC, Shifrin RY, Grishaw EK, Liu K, Gelfand DW (1994) Virtual colonoscopy (abstract). Radiology 193:446
3. Fishman EK (1998) Virtual Endoscopy. In: Fishman EK, Brook Jeffrey R Jr. (eds) Spiral CT: principles, techniques and clinical applications, 2nd edn. Lippincott-Raven, Philadelphia, pp 310–312
4. Vining DJ, Gelfand DW, Bechtold RE et al. (1994) Technical feasibility of colon imaging with helical CT and virtual reality (abstract). AJR Am J Roentgenol 162:104
5. Vining DJ (1996) Virtual endoscopy: is it reality? Radiology 200:30–31
6. McFarland EG, Brink JA et al. (1997) Visualization of colorectal polyps with spiral CT colography: evaluation of processing parameters with perspective volume rendering. Radiology 205:701–707
7. Brink JA, Wang G, McFarland EG (2000) Optimal section spacing in single-detector helical CT. Radiology 214:575–578
8. Ogata I, Komohara Y et al. (1999) CT evaluation of gastric lesions with three-dimensional display and interactive virtual endoscopy: comparison with conventional barium study and endoscopy. AJR Am J Roentgenol 172:1263–1270
9. Laghi A, Pavone Pet al. (1999) Volume-rendered spiral CT colography: assessment of diagnostic accuracy in the evaluation of colo-rectal disorders. Eur Radiol 10 [Suppl 3]:182 (Scientific Session ECR 2000)
10. Laghi A, Pavone P. et al. (1999) Multislice spiral CT colography: technique optimization. Eur Radiol 10 [Suppl 3]:182 (Scientific Session ECR 2000)
11. Hu H, He HD, Foley WD, Fox SH (2000) Four multidetector-row helical CT: image quality and volume coverage speed. Radiology 215:55–62
12. Calhoun PS, Kuszyk BS et al. (1999) Three-dimensional volume-rendering of spiral CT data: theory and method. RadioGraphics 19:745–764
13. Napel S (1998) Principles and techniques of 3D spiral CT angiography. In: Fishman EK, Brook Jeffrey R Jr. (eds) Spiral CT: principles, techniques and clinical applications, 2nd edn. Lippincott-Raven, Philadelphia, pp 339–360
14. Beaulieu CF, Rubin GD (1998) Perspective rendering of spiral CT data: flying through and around normal and pathologic anatomy. In Fishman EK, Brook Jeffrey R Jr. (eds) Spiral CT: principles, techniques and clinical applications, 2nd edn. Lippincott-Raven, Philadelphia, pp 35–52
15. Rubin GD, Beaulieu CF et al. (1996) Perspective volume rendering of CT and MR images: applications for endoscopic imaging. Radiology 199:321–330
16. Beaulieu CF, Brooke Jeffrey R et al. (1999) Display modes for CT colonography; part II: blinded comparison of axial CT and virtual endoscopic and panoramic endoscopic volume-rendered studies. Radiology 212:203–212
17. Paik D, Beaulieu CF, Brooke Jeffrey R et al. (1998) Automated flight path planning for virtual endoscopy. Med Phys 25:629–637
18. Paik D, Beaulieu CF, Brooke Jeffrey R (1998) Virtual colonoscopy visualization modes using cylindrical and planar map projections: techniques and evaluation. Radiology 209:429
19. Rogalla P, Bender A, Bick U et al. (2000) Tissue transition projection (TTP) of the intestines. Eur Radiol 10:806–810
20. Rogalla P, Bender A, Schmidt E et al. (1999) Comparison of virtual colonoscopy and tissue transition projection (TTP) in colorectal cancer. Eur Radiol 9 [Suppl 1]:144

21. Hopper KD, Iyriboz AT, Wise SW et al. (2000) Mucosal detail at virtual reality: surface versus volume rendering. Radiology 214:517–522
22. Fletcher JG, Luboldt W (2000) CT colonography and MR colonography: current status, research directions and comparison. Eur Radiol 10:786–801
23. Chen SU, Lu DS, Hecht JR et al. (1999) CT colonography: value of scanning in both the supine and prone positions. AJR Am J Roentgenol 172:595–599
24. Sheppard DG, Iyer RB, Herron D et al. (1999) Subtraction CT colonography: feasibility in an animal model. Clinical Radiology 54:126–132
25. Hara AK, Johnson CD, Reed JE et al. (1997) Reducing data size and radiation dose for CT colonography. AJR Am J Roentgenol 168:1181–1184
26. Fenlon HM, Nunes DP, Schroy PC et al. (1999) A comparison of virtual and conventional colonoscopy for the detection of colorectal polyps. N Engl J Med 341:1496–1503
27. Springer P, Dessl A, Giacomuzzi M et al. (1997) Virtual computed gastroscopy: a new technique. Endoscopy 29:632–634
28. Rogalla P, Werner-Rustner M et al. (1998) Virtual endoscopy of the small bowel: phantom study and preliminary clinical results. Eur Radiol 8:563–567
29. Lee DH (1998) Three-dimensional imaging of the stomach by spiral CT. JCAT 22:52–58

Multislice Computed Tomography Colonography: Technique Optimization

Andrea Laghi, Valeria Panebianco, Carlo Catalano,
Riccardo Iannaccone, Filippo G. Assael, Sante Iori,
Roberto Passariello

Introduction

Computed tomography colonography (CTC) is a recently developed technique for the evaluation of colonic disorders, which has been obtaining a wide consensus among radiologists, gastroenterologists, and also patients, thanks to the interesting preliminary clinical results and the optimal compliance [1, 2, 3]. Results from the literature, even if obtained with heterogeneity of acquisition techniques depending on differences in CT scanner technology, report high accuracy in the identification of colonic lesions, particularly polyps. Sensitivity is approaching 100% for the identification of polypoid lesions larger than 1 cm [4, 5, 6]. Moreover, the technique presents a very good patient acceptance due to minimum discomfort during examination and the relatively low invasiveness, which is limited to bowel preparation and colonic distension.

Nevertheless, some problems are evident. These are represented by
1. large examination volumes with consequent relatively long breath holds,
2. reduced spatial resolution along the z-axis, potentially leading to image misinterpretation of small lesions, and
3. dose exposure, particularly important if considering CTC as a screening method, especially in young patients [7, 8].

The development of multi-detector technology provides the availability of spiral CT scanners four to eight times faster than single row equipment, which might have the potential to address the above-mentioned limitations. The aim of our study was to optimize scanning parameters for CTC with a multislice CT scanner, using a home-made colonic phantom. A preliminary clinical study was also performed.

Materials and Methods

In Vitro Study

A colonic phantom was built using a 34-cm long air-filled acrylic tube, with an 80-mm internal diameter, an 88-mm external diameter, and an 8-mm parietal width. The tube was filled with 12 plastiline polyps with diameters of 3 mm, 5 mm, 7 mm, and 10 mm, located on four parallel rows of three polyps each

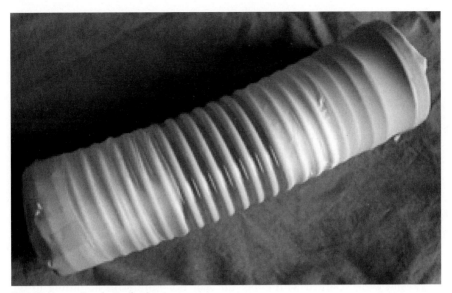

Fig. 1. Home-made colonic phantom

(Fig. 1). The mean density of the plastiline polyps was 800 HU. Before scanning, the colonic phantom was tightly closed at the extremities and was placed in a 40-cm square water-filled plastic box. A multislice CT SOMATOM Volume Zoom (Siemens, Erlangen, Germany) scanner, equipped with flying spot and adaptive array matrix was used. The colonic phantom was scanned, acquiring axial images (phantom parallel to the long axis of the moving table) and simulating the evaluation of the ascending and descending colon, 45° oblique images (phantom at 45° with respect to the long axis of the moving table), and sigmoid colon and colonic flexures.

Different scanning parameters were tested, using a 0.5-s gantry rotation time in each case:

1. Slice collimation 5 mm; slice width 7 mm; rotation feed 25 mm; reconstruction index 5 mm; acquisition time 10 s
2. Slice collimation 2.5 mm; slice width 3 mm; rotation feed 15 mm; reconstruction index 3 mm; acquisition time 14 s
3. Slice collimation 1 mm; slice width 1.25 mm; rotation feed 5 mm; reconstruction index 1 mm; acquisition time 30 s
4. Slice collimation 1 mm; slice width 1.25 mm; rotation feed 4 mm; reconstruction index 1 mm; acquisition time 30 s

The kilovolt peak [kV(p)] value was 120 for all protocols, whereas the milliamp values were 170 in protocol number (no.) 1, 130 in protocol no. 2, and 120 in protocols no. 3 and no. 4. Different milliamp values were used because of dose exposure-related problems and trying to maintain a less than 30-s acquisition time in each case.

In Vivo Study

A preliminary clinical study was performed in 12 patients (seven males and five females) who underwent multislice CTC. Patients presented with clinical indication for conventional colonoscopy (heme-positive stool, no. 4; altered bowel habit, no. 3; follow-up after hemicolectomy, no. 3) or after unsuccessful colonoscopy (no. 2).

Following standard oral colonoscopy preparation, consisting of 4 l of polyethylene glycol 4000 electrolyte solution [Isocolan; Bracco, Milan, Italy] taken the day before the examination, patients underwent CT study. Before image acquisition, an antiperistaltic drug (i.m. 20 mg of hyoscine butylbromine, Buscopan; Boehringer Ingelheim, Florence, Italy) was administered and, after placement of a rectal tube, the colon was gently insufflated with room air until maximum tolerance of the patient. The adequacy of the distension was assessed with an anteroposterior standard CT scout image. Further air insufflation was performed if required. Images were obtained during a single breath hold, with the patient in supine position. From the previous in vitro experience, two scanning protocols were chosen: no. 2 and no. 3 (for scanning parameters, see above).

Patients were scanned with either no. 2 or no. 3 protocols according to the following considerations:
1. duration of breath hold according to patient collaboration and age;
2. colon longitudinal extension, with the scan never exceeding a 30-s acquisition time; and
3. patient size, with larger patients scanned with a 3.0-mm slice width.

Duration of breath holds ranged from 14 s to 30 s, with patients instructed to start breathing quietly when the scan was at the level of the pelvis. From 280 s to 380 s, images were produced for each examination. When needed (i.e., in case of poor distension of segmentary colonic tracts or excessive retention of residual fluids), additional scans were obtained with the patient in a prone position. Due to dose considerations, no routine supine and prone scans were obtained in any of the cases. For each acquisition, dose exposure was calculated and never exceeded 9.12 mGy.

Image Processing

Once acquired, images were automatically transferred to our Picture Archiving and Communication System (Kodak, Milan, Italy) and successively downloaded to a dedicated workstation [Kayak PC workstation: two parallel kernel processors with a speed of 700 MHz each and 1024 Mb random access memory (RAM) memory; Hewlett Packard Palo Alto, Calif.]. Image elaboration was performed using Vitrea 2.0 (Vital Images, Fairfield, Iowa), a software with volume-rendering capabilities, where the user is asked to assign opacity values to pixels within a user-selected range of CT numbers. To generate three-dimensional (3D) endoluminal views, parameters were set to maximize the visualization of the air wall interface of the colonic phantom. Before image elaboration, no data segmentation was needed, and almost real-time generation of endoluminal views was performed.

Image Analysis

Images were interactively analyzed on a dedicated off-line workstation, and no print copy was obtained. A single radiologist, unaware of the number, size, and location of the simulated polyps, was asked to interactively review the 3D data sets, moving continuously through the slices. 2D axial images, 2D multiplanar reconstructions, and 3D endoluminal views were contemporarily available on a 17-inch monitor (43 cm). 2D images were analyzed using both lung (width 1000 HU; level –700 HU) and abdominal (width 360 HU; level 30 HU) windows.

Quantitative analysis consisted in the evaluation of the number of identified polyps and the polyp size along axial and longitudinal axes. Qualitative analysis consisted of evaluation of image artifacts and quality of 3D reconstructed images (step artifacts and polyp geometry deformation). Image quality was graded according to the following scale: optimal (no artifacts), good (mild artifacts with mild smoothing of polyp borders) and poor (severe artifacts and evident polyp distortion).

Results

Quantitative Analysis

In analysis of transverse scans, sensitivity of 100% was obtained for each polyp size and for each scanning protocol. With oblique scans, only a 3-mm polyp was missed when using protocol no. 1 parameters (sensitivity, 92%), whereas all the other polyps were identified on protocols no. 2, no. 3, and no. 4.

Measurement of polyp size was performed only for transverse acquisition. A good correlation between measured and real polyp size was observed when evaluating axial images, but polyp geometry distortion was observed when evaluating longitudinal reconstructions (see Table 1 for detailed results).

Table 1. Measurement of polyp size. Ax, axial axis; Long, longitudinal axis

	Polyp size 10 mm	7 mm	3 mm
Protocol 1			
Ax	10.7	7.4	3.4
Long	22.1	13.4	9.7
Protocol 2			
Ax	10.0	7.5	3.5
Long	16.2	11.2	7.1
Protocol 3			
Ax	9.8	7.2	3.5
Long	17.1	12.2	5.4
Protocol 4			
Ax	10.2	7.5	3.3
Long	15.7	11.7	5.1

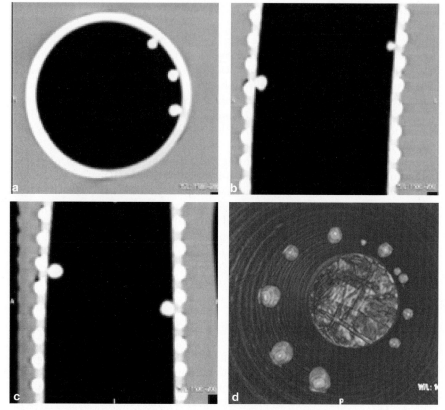

Fig. 2a–d. Images obtained from protocol number 1 (axial acquisition with thin collimation, 1 mm). **a** Axial plane showing clear identification of three 1-cm polyps. Sagittal (**b**) and coronal (**c**) reformatted images showing no significant deformation of polyp size and no step artifacts. **d** A three-dimensional endoluminal view shows polys inside the phantom with preservation of morphology and size

Qualitative Analysis

Image quality was graded as optimal for protocols no. 3 and no. 4, where no major artifacts were evident in both axial and oblique acquisitions, and no significant smoothing of the borders of polyps was observed in 3D reconstructions (Fig. 2 a–d and Fig. 3 a–c). In protocol no. 2, quality was graded as optimal when analyzing transverse scans and as good when analyzing oblique scans. Protocol no. 1 was graded as good on transverse scans and as poor on oblique scans (Fig. 4 a–d and Fig. 5 a–d).

Patients' Results

Images of diagnostic quality were obtained in all of the cases. No artifacts secondary to respiratory motion were observed. The quality of the 3D reconstructions

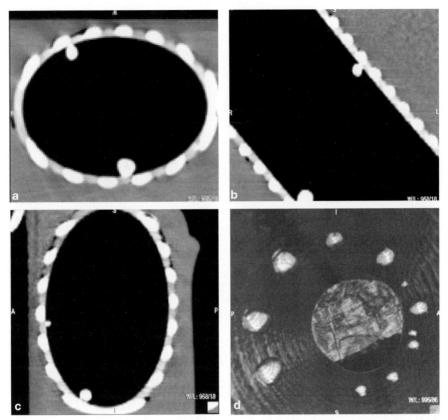

Fig. 3a–d. Images obtained from protocol number 1 (oblique acquisition with thin collimation, 1 mm). Compared with previous axial acquisition, no significant differences in polyp size are visible on axial (**a**), sagittal (**b**), and coronal (**c**) planes, although minor step artifacts are evident. On a three-dimensional endoluminal view, slight deformation of polyp borders is evident (**d**)

was graded as optimal for protocol no. 3 and as good for protocol no. 2. When using protocol no. 2, minor step artifacts were present, especially when observing endoluminal views at higher magnification and on oblique planes. In this preliminary experience, two colonic carcinomas and three 10-mm polyps were detected (two when using protocol no. 2 and one with protocol no. 3).

Discussion

Since 1994, when Vining [9] proposed a new technique for colonic evaluation based on computed elaboration of 3D CT data sets, named as virtual colonoscopy, several technical progresses occurred. They involved both scanner technology and computer systems, leading to shorter examination time and better quality of 3D reconstructed images. The former were represented by the evolution of spiral CT equipment in terms of gantry rotation time with the develop-

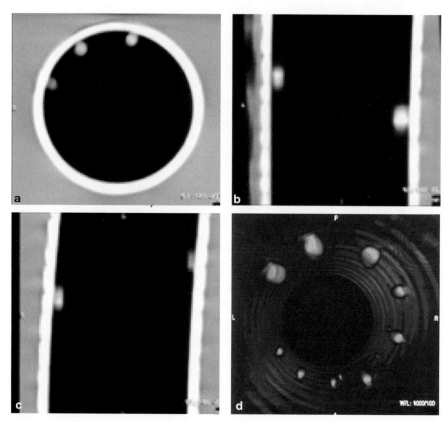

Fig. 4a–d. Images obtained from protocol number 4 (axial acquisition with thick collimation, 5 mm). a Axial plane showing clear identification of two 1-cm polyps. Sagittal (**b**) and coronal (**c**) reformatted images showing deformation of polyp size and morphology along the z-axis. **d** A three-dimensional endoluminal view shows only mild deformation of morphology and size of polyps with smoothing borders compared with thin collimation acquisition

ment of sub-second scanners and in detector technology, leading to multi-slice equipment. The computer systems included rapid improvements in terms of computational power, providing more powerful and, at the same time, cheaper workstations for 3D data management, which were able to support complex and heavy software for 3D reconstructions, such as volume-rendering [10]. Technical progresses allowed optimal and reproducible clinical results to be reached, even if obtained with heterogeneity of acquisition techniques, depending on differences in CT scanner technology.

In terms of diagnostic accuracy, a 100% sensitivity in the detection of large colonic lesions (>2 cm) and polyps larger than 1 cm in diameter is now assumed [11, 12, 13]. The identification of smaller polyps, especially when less than 5 mm in diameter, remains as a diagnostic problem. Poor results in the identification of small lesions might be attributed to low spatial resolution of CT images, especially along the z-axis, due to pitch restrictions.

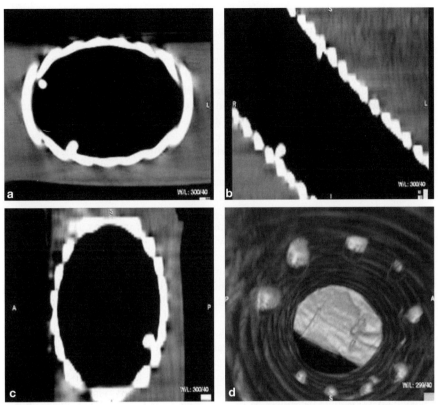

Fig. 5a–d. Images obtained from protocol number 4 (oblique acquisition with thick collimation, 5 mm). **a** Axial plane showing clear identification of two 1-cm polyps. Sagittal (**b**) and coronal (**c**) reformatted images showing severe artifacts and elongation of polyp size. **d** A three-dimensional endoluminal view shows severe artifacts with deformation of morphology and size of polyps; borders are severely smoothed

The second problem of CTC is represented by the relatively long acquisition time and the consequent long breath hold period. This is due to the fact that a large volume coverage is needed. The mean length of the acquisition to cover the entire colon within a single spiral CT acquisition is 40 cm. Single acquisition is now considered mandatory in order to avoid misregistration artifacts typically evident on images from preliminary studies performed with older scanners [14, 15]. These two problems are strictly interconnected with the increase of spatial resolution limited by the breath hold period and vice versa. Moreover, both of them are also related with dose administration to the patient.

The development of multi-detector technology provides the availability of spiral CT scanners four to eight times faster than single row equipment, which might address the technical limitations pointed out above. In fact, multi-detector spiral CT scanners provide an almost isotropic resolution if using thin collimation and image reconstruction index, with the generation of high quality multi-planar reconstructions and 3D endoscopic views. Only a minimal distortion of the geometry of both large and small lesions was observed when evaluating thin collimation protocols.

In our experience, lesion identification was possible in all of the cases for any lesion size, except one small lesion was missed on the thicker collimation protocol with oblique acquisition; severe artifacts were also observed. A possible limitation of our study was the very high density of plastiline used for producing simulated polyps. It was much higher than the tissue density of real polypoid lesions. This situation might lead to an easier identification of polypoid lesions. Further studies with simulated polyps with lower density values are in progress.

Fast multi-slice acquisition may be used for increasing either the speed of acquisition or the longitudinal spatial resolution. In fact, it is possible to obtain fast acquisition to cover the entire abdomen from the diaphragm to the anal canal within 15 s and still maintain an optimal spatial resolution, thanks to the higher pitch values to be employed on multislice CT scanners. As a consequence, we were able to study the entire colon with a protocol (3-mm collimation) comparable with the techniques implemented on single slice scanners and within an acquisition time of around one-third compared with previous studies. This leads to a shorter examination time, which is more comfortable for the less cooperative and older patients, and a consequent reduction in terms of dose exposure due to reduced a acquisition time.

It was also possible to develop protocols with 1-mm collimation, resulting in almost isotropic voxels and optimal quality of both multi-planar 2D reformations and 3D endoluminal views. In this case, a decrease of the milliamp value is necessary in order to reduce dose exposure. An important consideration concerning the choice of the adequate acquisition technique is related to the workload. A major difference is present between 3-mm and 1-mm protocols, with the latter generating a considerably higher number of images. The management of 300–400 images is not easy, both in terms of capacity of picture archiving and communication systems (PACS) and in speed of reconstruction and elaboration of 3D images on dedicated workstations. More powerful computer processors and the need of longer image reconstruction time for image editing are requirements which have to be considered when evaluating the cost-effectiveness of the procedure. Moreover, when dealing with patients, different considerations need to be taken into account concerning also the patient's clinical conditions (cooperation for longer breath holds) and age (dose exposure). The real clinical benefit of high-resolution protocols needs to be evaluated through dedicated studies in terms of lesion identification.

In conclusion, multi-detector technology offers new possibilities in terms of techniques to be implemented for CT evaluation of the colon, providing faster acquisition for covering the entire volume and/or increase of spatial resolution along the longitudinal axis. The choice between faster and very high-resolution protocols needs to be defined by further clinical studies.

References

1. Vining DJ (1999) Virtual colonoscopy. Semin Ultrasound CT MR 20:56–60
2. Fenlon HM, Ferrucci JT (1997) Virtual colonoscopy: what will the issues be? AJR Am J Roentgenol 169:453–458
3. Forbes GM, Mendelson RM (2000) Patient acceptance of virtual colonoscopy. Endoscopy 32:274–275
4. Fenlon HM, Nunes DP, Schroy PC, Barish MA, Clarke PD, Ferrucci JT (1999) A comparison of virtual and conventional colonoscopy for the detection of colorectal polyps. N Engl J Med 341:1496–1503
5. Hara AK, Johnson CD, Reed JE, et al. (1997) Detection of colorectal polyps with CT colonography: initial assessment of sensitivity and specificity. Radiology 205:59–65
6. Johnson CD, Hara AK, Reed JE (1997) Computed tomographic colonography (virtual colonoscopy): a new method for detecting colorectal neoplasms. Endoscopy29:454–461
7. McFarland EG, Brink JA (1999) Helical CT colonography (virtual colonoscopy): the challenge that exists between advancing technology and generalizability. AJR Am J Roentgenol 173:549–559
8. Rigatus H, Marchal G, Baert AL, et al. (1990) Spiral scanning and the influence of the reconstruction algorithm on image quality. J Comput Assist Tomogr 14:675–682
9. Vining DJ, Gelfand DW, Bechtold RE, Scharling ES, Grishaw EK, Shifrin RY (1994) Technical feasibility of colon imaging with helical CT and virtual reality (abstract). AJR Am J Roentgenol 162[suppl]:104
10. Rubin GD, Beaulieu CF, Argiro V, Ringl H, et al. (1996) Perspective volume rendering of CT and MR images: applications for endoscopic imaging. Radiology 199:321–330
11. Fenlon HM, Nunes DP, Clarke PD, Ferrucci JT (1998) Colorectal neoplasm detection using virtual colonoscopy: a feasibility study. Gut 43:806–811
12. Fenlon HM, McAneny DB, Nunes DP, Clarke PD, Ferrucci JT (1999) Occlusive colon carcinoma: virtual colonoscopy in the preoperative evaluation of the proximal colon. Radiology 210:423–428
13. Johnson CD, Ahlquist DA (1999) Computed tomography colonography (virtual colonoscopy) a new method of colorectal screening. Gut44:301–305
14. Rigatus H, Marchal G, Baert AL, et al. (1990) Spiral scanning and the influence of the reconstruction algorithm on image quality. J Comput Assist Tomogr 14:675–682
15. Beaulieu CF, Napel S, Daniel BL, Ch'en IY, Rubin GD, Johnstone IM, Jeffrey RB Jr (1998) Detection of colonic polyps in a phantom model: implications for virtual colonoscopy data acquisition. J Comput Assist Tomogr 22:656–663

Subject Index

abdominal aorta and / or thoracic aneurysm or dissection 128
abdomen multislice CT applications 179–187
acetabular fractures 40
adaptive
– array detector (AAD) 9, 10
– imaging reconstruction 119
Agatston score 86, 102
– method 102
algorithm 360 / 180° 4
aneurysms
– cerebral 62
– left ventricular 108
– popliteal artery aneurysm 137
– thoracic and / or abdominal aorta aneurysm or dissection 128
angiography
– coronary MSCT angiography 104, 121
– CT angiography (CTA) 5, 7, 25–27
angioscopy, virtual 121, 122
aortic stents 41
array detector, adaptive (AAD) 9, 10
artery / arteries / arterial
– arterial occlusive lesions 61
– carotid arteries 26
– CT angiogram, arterial and venous phases 127
– obstructive arterial disease, lower extremities 134
– peripheral arteries 137
– phase 200
– popliteal artery aneurysm 137
AVMs, brain 63

beam collimation 8–10
brain
– AVMs 63
– tumors 64
breath hold scanning 16
bronchial carcinoma screening 154
bronchiectases 148
bronchogenic carcinoma 151, 153

bronchoscopy, virtual 47–59, 155
– indications 48
bypass, coronary 91
– grafts 91, 107

CAD (coronary artery disease) 118
calcified / calcifications
– calcified plaque 113
– coronary (*see there*) 16, 91, 102, 106
calcium
– coronary (*see there*) 102, 103, 106, 118
– scoring 120
calibration standards 85
capillary space 30
cardiac
– CT imaging 16, 79–89
– – quality assurance 84–86
– function / functional anaylsis 116, 118–124, 123
– MSCT 79–89
– prospective cardiac triggering 79, 118, 119
– retrospective cardiac gating 79
cardio-CT, potential of 90–97
carotid arteries 26
cerebral aneurysms 62
cervical three-dimensional CTA 59–64
chest CT, radiation exposure 169–176
cholesteatoma 69, 72
collimation / collimators 7, 195
– beam collimation 8–10
– width of collimators 126
colonography, CT (CTC) 216–225
colonoscopy, virtual 44, 210–212
combi scan 147
contrast / contrast media (c.m.) 196, 197
– c.m. administration 22, 27, 28
– delivery parameters 4
– enhancement 22, 28
– high-contrast organs 173
– intravenous administration of the contrast agents 137
coronary
– angiography 104

- arteries / artery disease (CAD) 79, 118,
  118–124
- - imaging of 111
- atherosclerosis in MSCT 98–109
- bypass (*see there*) 91, 107
- calcium 102, 103
- - detection 106
- - quantitative assessment of /
    quantification 102, 106, 120
- - scoring 79, 80, 120
- calcifications 16, 91, 102
- - screening 106
- imaging 19
- - direct coronal and sagittal imaging 125
- stents 107, 108
coverage 4
craniocervical junction 73
craniofacial surgery 40
CT / CT imaging
- cardiac CT imaging (*see there*) 16, 79–89
- CT angiography (CTA) 5, 7, 25–27
- - arterial and venous phases 127
- - cervical three-dimensional 59–64
- - fast high-resolution CT angiography of
    peripheral vessels 134–142
- - intracranial three-dimensional
    59–64
- CT enhancement 30
- CTDI (CT dose index) 170
- electron beam CT (*see* EBCT) 81, 90,
  91, 98
- HRCT (high-resolution CT) 170
- low dose CT 151
- multislice CT (*see* MSCT) 37, 59–64,
  65–74, 98–109, 121
- potential of cardio-CT 90–97
CTC (colonography CT) 216–225
CTDI (CT dose index) 170

data glove 51
dissection, thoracic and / or abdominal
  aortic aneurysm or dissection 128
documentation 5, 6, 147, 173
- examination protocol 6
- high-resolution protocol
  (thin collimation) 146
- high-speed protocol (fast) 147
- low-dose protocol 173
- MSCT protocol, liver and pancreas 199
- single-slice)
  nephron-sparing protocol 182
- multislice)
  nephron-sparing protocol 184
dose / dosage
- effective dose 171
- low dose CT 151, 171

EBCT (electron beam CT) 81, 90, 91, 98
- coronary atherosclerosis 98
- ECG-triggering in 91
ECG
- ECG-based reconstruction algorithm 79
- ECG gating 16, 94
- - retrospective 16, 99, 100, 111, 118, 119
- ECG-triggering 16, 90
- - EBCT 91
- - prospective 16, 99, 118, 119
- - sequential scanning 98
embolism, pulmonary 157–168, 175
endoluminal aortic stent 50
endoscopy / endoscopic
- endoscopic views 18
- virtual 37, 43–49, 204–215
endotracheal stent planning 49
examination protocol 6
exposure duration 4
extravascular space 30

fast high-resolution CT angiography of
  peripheral vessels 134–142
fibrosis, idiopathic pulmonary fibrosis 149
focused studies 5

Gantry rotation speed 4
gastroscopy, virutal 212, 213

heart
- arteries 79
- rate 20
hematuria 189–191
high-resolution protocol (thin collimation)
  146
high-speed protocol (fast) 147
histiocytosis X 68
HRCT (high-resolution CT) 170

image, noice 3
- sharpness 4
implants, standard 51
interstitial spaces 30
intestinal ischemia 128
intracranial
- lesion 68
- three-dimensional CTA 59–64
intraorbital lesion 68
intravascular
- space 30
- ultrasound 105
iodine concentration 23, 25, 30
isotropic
- data sets 38
- imaging 8, 11
- resolution 16, 17
IVU (intravenous urography) 189

kVp 4

left ventricular aneurysm 108
lipid-rich plaques, non-calcified 122
liver 195–199
– enhancement strategies 197, 198
– MSCT protocol 199
low dose
– CT 151, 171
– protocol 173
lower extremities, obstructive arterial
  disease 134
lung
– cancer screening 173
– diffuse lung disease 155
– nodules 153
– – nodule characterization 153
– parenchyma 145–156
lymph node staging 154

mA 4
marching cubes algorithm 39
max. intensity projections (MIP) 40, 126
metastatic nodule detection 173
milliamps 173
MIP (maximum intensity projection) 40,
  126
MSCT (multislice CT) 10, 11, 37, 59–64,
  79–89, 98–109, 121
– abdominal multislice CT applications
  179–187
– advantages 10
– cardiac 79–89
– cervical and intracranial three-dimensional 59–64
– coronary
– – atherosclerosis in MSCT 98–109
– – MSCT angiography 104, 121
– liver 195–199
– pancreas (see there) 195, 197–202
– pulmonary embolism 157–168
– skull base 65–74
– transaxial 10
– urinary tract 188–194
mucocele 65
multi-planar
– reconstruction 38, 39
– reformation (MPRs) 11, 37, 180
myocardial infarction 108

nasopharyngeal carcinoma 70
nephrectomy, partial 181
nephron-sparing surgery 181
– single-sclice
  nephron-sparing protocol 182
– multislice
  nephron-sparing protocol 184

nodule
– characterization 153
– metastatic nodule detection 173
non-calcified plaques
– lipid-rich 18, 104, 105, 122

obstructive arterial disease,
  lower extremities 134
oncologic patient 5
oncology tumor staging 127
organ transplant evaluation 127
Osler's disease 150
osmolarity 23
otitis media, chronic 69

pancreas 195, 197–202
– 3D imgaing 201
– enhancement strategies 197, 198
– limitations of MSCT 201
– MSCT protocol 199
partial volume averaging effect 4
petrous bone 69, 71
phase shift artifact 114
pitch (p) 170, 174, 195, 196
– factor 146, 147
– table feed speed (pitch) 4
pixel 3
plaques
– calcified 113
– non-calcified 18, 104, 105
– – lipid-rich plaques 122
polyps, simulated 219
popliteal
– artery aneurysm 137
– entrapment 141
portal venous phase 200
protocol (see documentation) 5, 6, 147, 173
pulmonary
– embolism, multislice CT 157–168, 175
– fibrosis, idiopathic 149
– fissures 152
– hypertension (PH) 163
– vasculature 26
– vessels 154, 155

quality assurance 84–86

radiation
– dose 3
– exposure 190
– – chest CT 169–176
raw data set, secondary 148
ray sum display 209
real time visualization of volume data
  125–133
reconstruction
– adaptive imaging 119

– algorithm 4
– increment 4
– interval 195, 196
– kernel 5
– segmented 119
renal mass evaluation 192
rigid bone tissue 51
rotation
– speed, Gantry rotation speed 4
– time 7, 79

sagittal imaging 125
scan / scanning
– breath hold scanning 16
– combi scan 147
– scan timing 28, 79, 197
screening
– for colorectal cancer 44
– coronary calcifications 106
secondary raw data set 148
shaded surface display (surface rendering)
    39–41, 206
skull base 65–75
– fracture of 67
slice
– thickness 4
– width 14
small bowel 213
soft tissues 51
SSD (surface shaded display) 138
standard implants 51
stents
– aortic 41, 50
– coronary 107, 108
– endotracheal stent planning 49
surface rendering (shaded surface display)
    39–41, 206
surgical simulation 49–54
survey studies 5

table feed speed (see also pitch) 4
technical parameters 5
thin collimation
    (high-resolution protocol) 146
thoracic and / or abdominal aortic
    aneurysm or dissection 128

three-dimensional imaging 37–56
threshold value 40
thrombosis, deep venous 166, 167
tissue transition projection (TTP) 209
tracheobronchial system 155
trauma 5

urinary tract 188–194
urography, intravenous (IVU) 189
user-selectable parameters 4

vascular
– persistence 23
– spaces 30
venous
– phases
– – CT angiogram 127
– – intravenous administration of the
        contrast agents 137
– – portal venous phase 200
– thrombosis, deep venous 166, 167
vessels
– peripheral, fast high-resolution CT
    angiography 134–142
– pulmonary 154
virtual
– angioscopy 121, 122
– bronchoscopy 47–59, 155
– colonoscopy 44, 210–212
– endoscopy (VE) 37, 43–49, 204–215
– gastroscopy 212, 213
viscosity 23
volume
– averaging effect, partial 4
– coverage 8, 16
– real time visualization, volume data
    125–133
– rendering (VRs) 11, 41–43, 138, 150, 180,
    207, 208

width of the collimators 126

X-ray tube 5

Z-axis resolution 6

Printing: Druckhaus Beltz, Hemsbach
Binding: Buchbinderei Schäffer, Grünstadt